P9-AZX-117

# The ALLERGY SOLUTION
# for DOGS

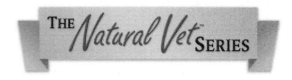

# THE Natural Vet SERIES

# The ALLERGY SOLUTION for DOGS

•

## NATURAL AND CONVENTIONAL THERAPIES TO EASE DISCOMFORT AND ENHANCE YOUR DOG'S QUALITY OF LIFE

*Shawn Messonnier, D.V.M.*

PRIMA PETS
AN IMPRINT OF PRIMA PUBLISHING
3000 LAVA RIDGE COURT • ROSEVILLE, CALIFORNIA 95661
(800) 632-8676 • WWW.PRIMALIFESTYLES.COM

**DISCLAIMER:** While the Publisher and the author have designed this book to provide up-to-date information in regard to the subject matter covered, readers should be aware that medical information is constantly evolving. The information presented herein is of a general nature and is not intended as a substitute for professional medical advice. Readers should consult with a qualified veterinarian for specific instructions on the treatment and care of their pet. The author and Prima Publishing shall have neither liability nor responsibility to any person or entity with respect to any loss, damage, or injury caused or alleged to be caused directly or indirectly by the information contained in this book.

THE NATURAL VET series and PRIMA PETS are trademarks of Prima Communications, Inc. The Prima colophon is a trademark of Prima Communications Inc., registered with the United States Patent and Trademark Office.

All products mentioned in this book are trademarks of their respective companies.

Library of Congress Cataloging-in-Publication Data
Messonnier, Shawn.
    The allergy solution for dogs : natural and conventional therapies to ease discomfort and enhance your dog's quality of life / Shawn Messonnier.
        p.   cm.
    ISBN 0-7615-2672-2
    1. Allergy in dogs.  I. Title
SF992.A44 M47 2000
636.7'089697—dc21                                                   00-029132

00 01 02 03 HH 10 9 8 7 6 5 4 3 2 1
Printed in the United States of America

**How to Order**
Single copies may be ordered from Prima Publishing, 3000 Lava Ridge Court, Roseville, CA 95661; telephone (800) 632-8676 ext. 4444. Quantity discounts are also available. On your letterhead, include information concerning the intended use of the books and the number of books you wish to purchase.

**Visit us online at www.primalifestyles.com**

# CONTENTS

# FOREWORD

THE PAST FIVE years have seen a huge outpouring of interest by pet owners and veterinarians about the practice of holistic veterinary medicine. Just as people have been able to experience the benefits first hand of holistic and natural approaches to their own health, they naturally want to convey these same benefits to their four-legged family members.

Healthy family interactions play a large role in promoting the health and wellness of all family members (including pets). Dysfunctional family dynamics can likewise promote illness and chronic disease in our pets. To better promote the health of the animal and the family that it lives with, the holistic veterinarian, as part of this holistic process, tries to make a better "fit" between the animal and its family. This healthier connection will contribute to optimal health and happiness within the family unit.

Holistic veterinarians try to follow the Hippocratic Oath which states: "Above All, Do No Harm." Holistic vets try to avoid the unnecessary use of drugs and surgeries if they are not needed to improve the animal's health. Vaccinations, for example, although helpful in preventing certain epidemic and epizootic diseases, may not be necessary every year. (Only the rabies vaccine is required by law in every state.) Duration of immunity studies are now being completed which are demonstrating that vaccinations given early in the life of the animal (by 12 weeks of age) may have a protectiveness that lasts for many, many years, if not for the life of the animal.

Another commonly held assumption that holistic veterinarians question includes the wisdom of feeding nothing but commercial dog food for the life of the pet. It has been recognized in recent years that commercial pet foods are overly processed, laden with adulterants, and made from poor quality, raw materials, much of which have been condemned for human consumption. In my own clinical practice of 18 years, I have found no greater healing tool for my patients than to take them off a commercial diet and switch them (slowly and gradually!) to a fresh, wholesome (and in many cases), raw food diet.

This very complete and well-written book by Dr. Shawn Messonnier will provide you with a well-balanced approach to keeping your pets healthy. I agree with his perspective that holistic veterinary health care is an integration of the best of conventional medicine and the best of alternative medicine. Messonnier does not "throw the baby out with the bath water" in promoting this perspective, rather he promotes a commonsense, integrated, and complementary approach to animal health care.

THE NATURAL VET™ series by Dr. Shawn Messonnier, will be a valuable addition to the natural health care section of your library, whether you are a "pet parent" wanting to give your four-legged family member a more natural upbringing or a veterinarian wanting to learn more about these useful and emerging therapies. As a veterinarian, I have found that my clients have appreciated my adding these new "natural" tools to my practice bag. THE NATURAL VET™ series will join the many other fine books available at my veterinary clinic.

*Robert J. Silver, D.V.M, M.S.*

# PREFACE

I AM A CONVENTIONAL doctor by training, an Aggie from the Lone Star State. I graduated in 1987 from Texas A&M University with a doctorate of veterinary medicine and, in 1991, opened Paws & Claws Animal Hospital, the first referral hospital for dogs, cats, and exotic pets in Plano, Texas.

After using conventional treatments for several years, I became convinced that many pets that were not improving with lifelong use of conventional medications might improve if some type of alternative was available. This desire to improve the quality of my patients' lives led me to become adept at treating pets with a variety of complementary therapies. Due to the success of this idea, I created the Acupuncture and Holistic Animal Health Care Center, the only hospital in the area to offer both conventional and complementary therapies for dogs and cats.

Now, in addition to practicing medicine, I spread the word of holistic health care for pets as a regular columnist for the *Dallas Morning News* and the *Wylie News*. For two years, I hosted Fox Television's "4 Your Pets" pet care show. I serve on the board of the prestigious international journal *Veterinary Forum* and I am also founder and editor-in-chief of *Exotic Pet Practice,* the only monthly international publication devoted to the care of exotic pets. Each month I reach over half a million pet owners as the holistic columnist for both *Dog Fancy* and *Cat Fancy* magazines. I also serve as a consultant to Our Pets, a leading manufacturer of natural pet products, and am the holistic veterinarian for www.planet-pets.com.

This book, *The Allergy Solution for Dogs,* is part of a brand-new series of health guides called THE NATURAL VET™. With this exciting project I hope to show you ways to care for your pets using safe, natural, alternative treatments for a variety of medical conditions.

As a speaker, consultant, and writer, I teach veterinarians and pet owners around the world how holistic methods can reduce the cost of veterinary care and help pets live longer, healthier lives. I challenge everyone I work with to be the best they can be and to rise above any challenges they may face, and I am committed to providing the best health care possible for my patients.

*A note about natural supplements:*

Throughout the book I have mentioned a number of natural supplements that can assist the pet with allergies. I have tried to be as objective as possible, and have tried to refrain from promoting any particular products. Still, every doctor has favorites that have worked best in his or her practice, and I have pointed these out when necessary. Since there are many products available, I encourage you to work with your doctor to find the best products that are most suitable for your pet.

# ACKNOWLEDGMENTS

THE *ALLERGY SOLUTION For Dogs* is the second book in the THE NATURAL VET™ series. I am happy to be working with the fine folks at Prima Publishing, including my editors, Lorna Eby and Libby Larson, and publisher, Ben Dominitz. Their vision and acceptance of my idea for a holistic series was instrumental in getting this book into your hands.

A big thanks to all holistic doctors for sharing their ideas with me and with the profession through their books and clinical articles. Your desire to do what is best for our pets is appreciated by all.

A special thanks to Dr. Christina Chambreau for her help with the section on homeopathy.

Drs. Joseph Kandel and David Sudderth wrote *The Arthritis Solution* (for people). Their great book served as a guide and template for the books in THE NATURAL VET™ series. Thank you!

Thank you to God for the talent and drive to do all I desire.

Finally, as always, a big "thanks, hugs, and kisses" to Sandy and Erica. Your support means a lot!

# INTRODUCTION

ALTHOUGH THERE ARE many causes of itchiness in dogs, the most common is a genetic inflammatory disease called atopic (allergic) dermatitis, often called skin allergies. *The Allergy Solution for Dogs* deals with the treatment of this allergic condition in a holistic way. Unlike other holistic pet books, this book is an objective assessment of the most commonly recommended therapies—both conventional and complementary—for dogs with atopic dermatitis.

This book explores all these treatment approaches so that you, the pet owner, working with your veterinarian, can determine the best course of action. The book is not meant to replace a visit to a qualified veterinary clinic. There are many potentially serious causes of itchiness in dogs and a proper diagnosis is vital for the recovery of your pet. Use the information in this book as a starting point of discussion between you and your veterinarian.

## THE HOLISTIC MINDSET

YOU MAY BE surprised to find a chapter on conventional therapies for treating allergies in a holistic book, but the two are not contradictory. "Holistic" means "looking at the whole pet and doing what is in the pet's best interests." In order to be open to what is best for your dog, doctors and pet owners alike must develop what I call a holistic mindset. "Holistic care" refers to a way of thinking. The holistic doctor and owner view the dog in its entirety, rather than just blindly focusing on a set of problems or signs and symptoms.

The holistic mindset considers all options, and then chooses those that are best for your pet. This means that occasionally a conventional medicine might be needed to help relieve the itching and inflammation that dogs with allergic dermatitis suffer. As long as we use these conventional therapies in an intelligent way, we are acting holistically. In *The Allergy Solution for Dogs,* you will learn how to help your dog with both conventional therapies as well as more natural methods.

> With every treatment we contemplate using, we must ask, "Is this best for the dog?"

By changing our thought processes and becoming more holistic, everyone, especially our pets, benefits. Simply put, we must be open-minded and always put the dog's interests first. With every treatment we contemplate using, we must ask, "Is this best for the dog?" Having a holistic attitude means that doctors and owners refuse to focus just on the problem at hand, but instead prefer to focus on total wellness for the pet. The goal of holistic care is disease prevention. As a holistic doctor, I prefer to "treat the pet" rather than, at best, treat a disease or, at worst, treat signs and symptoms. Ultimately, the pet benefits from this way of care.

# Understand Your Treatment Options

When it comes to treating an allergic dog, you have quite a few options. The reason for the large number of choices is that there is truly no one "best" solution for every dog's problem. I believe that each pet is an individual, and must be treated as such. In my private practice, I discuss this philosophy with owners right from the start. I explain that what worked for the last allergic dog I treated may not work for their pet. Each owner is different as well, with different wants and a different budget. Some pet owners want to do everything possible— money is no object—and they have the time and interest plus a cooperative animal. This allows us to experiment and try a number of unique approaches. Other people opt for a bit less. They do not feel comfortable with alternative ideas, and may not mind their pet taking conventional medications for the long haul. Still others decide not to give their animals any medications and choose only natural alternative therapies.

Alternative therapy means any therapy that is an alternative to conventional medical treatment. This includes nutritional supplements, herbal medicine, homeopathy, and acupuncture, to name a few common ones. The term "complementary therapy" is often used interchangeably with alternative therapy, but this practice is not really correct. "Alternative" implies "something other than." "Complementary therapy" implies that the chosen treatment is "complementing" the standard treatment, and not necessarily replacing it.

Since most holistic doctors are open to both forms of treatment, the preferred term "complementary therapy" means that our treatment, such as acupuncture or homeopathy, is used in conjunction with and complements the conventional medical therapy that we may also prescribe. "Natural care" refers to using treatments other than conventional drug therapies.

# COMPLEMENTARY THERAPIES AND RESEARCH

ONE OF THE difficulties in writing a book discussing complementary therapies for pets is trying to find good research showing that these therapies actually work. Unlike the volumes of research data on conventional drug therapies, there just isn't as much data available on complementary therapies. The basic reason for this is financial. The company doing the study (usually the manufacturer of the drug) must be prepared to spend a lot of money—often hundreds of thousands and even millions of dollars—to run the kind of double-blind, placebo-controlled study considered the gold standard of research in conventional medicine. In order to spend this large sum of money, the company must have money for research and, to justify spending it, must expect to be able to recoup the investment plus a nice profit in the future.

> Alternative therapy means any therapy that is an alternative to conventional medical treatment.

Most companies that manufacture complementary remedies do not have this kind of capital. Even if they did, the chance of making enough profit from their product often does not exist. In addition, since many complementary remedies are natural products, such as herbs, they cannot be patented.

Without a patent, there is no financial incentive to run the study. Homeopathic remedies, another common complementary therapy, cannot be patented either. Unfortunately, this means that we don't have many good double-blind, placebo-controlled studies to use to back up our recommendations for treating allergic pets with complementary therapies.

Why are double-blind, placebo-controlled studies considered the gold standard? In this type of study, neither the doctor nor the patient (in this case the pet owner) knows if the treatment being administered is the "active agent" or the placebo. This lack of knowledge on the part of both doctor and owner is why such a study is termed "double-blind." Since there are always some patients who get better on a placebo, this type of study uses a placebo so that the number of pets who respond to the "active agent" can be statistically compared with the number of pets responding to the placebo.

This kind of study is ideal to "prove" or "disprove" that a certain recommended therapy works, and is always done to get government approval for a new drug. Since most complementary therapies do not have the benefit of this type of study, they are open to a lot of criticism from conventional doctors.

The evidence I consider for the complementary therapies I use and recommend often comes from my own clinical experience and the experience of other established holistic veterinarians. I know that these therapies work because we have been using them for years (as have veterinarians before us) and I can see the results. While this anecdotal evidence may not be as good as the double-blind, placebo-controlled research, often it is all that is available. A combination of therapies is most often the most effective and that makes it difficult to test any one of the herbs and supplements given to the pet because they work together. Many of the recommended therapies in *The Allergy Solution for Dogs* fall into this category.

The final source of my research on complementary therapies for allergic pets is extrapolation from the scientific literature on humans. In many instances throughout this book, I mention approaches that research either suggests may work on people or has proved that it works. While there are no guarantees, nor should we automatically extrapolate from the human literature and apply it to pets, if a treatment works for people, it may work on animals. Therefore, I have included these therapy options for you to discuss with your doctor.

# THE PARTNERSHIP APPROACH

THE GOAL OF this book is to make you an informed consumer of veterinary information so that you become an active participant in the care of your itchy dog. By informing you of all the possible causes of itching and what you can expect at a veterinary visit, I hope to prepare you to know what symptoms to look for in your dog and what questions to ask your dog's doctor so that your pet receives a proper diagnosis. By offering you options in both conventional and complementary treatment for allergies, I hope to enable you to establish a holistic approach that best serves your pet. By providing diet and allergy prevention techniques, I hope to assist you in becoming a partner in your dog's care. Bu working together, you and your veterinarian can help your pet avoid skin allergies and enjoy a wonderful, itch-free life.

# · 1 ·

# Understanding Allergies

I F YOUR DOG is scratching regularly without signs of skin lesions, chances are he has an allergy. Atopic (allergic) dermatitis is among the most common skin diseases seen in dogs. If you are interested in holistic pet care to treat this condition, you must find a veterinarian who shares this mindset and keeps up-to-date with research on complementary treatment options. But first you must determine that your dog's itchiness is indeed caused by atopic (allergic) dermatitis.

## GET A PROPER DIAGNOSIS

THE TECHNICAL TERM for skin allergies is atopic dermatitis, also called atopy. Atopy is a genetic inflammatory disease in which the dog becomes sensitized to environmental protein stimuli called allergens (pollens, molds, ragweeds, house dust mites). In non-allergic dogs, these allergens do not cause problems. In allergic or atopic dogs, these allergens produce the clinical signs so commonly seen. Most pets are diagnosed with atopic dermatitis based upon clinical signs, history, and response to corticosteroids or antihistamines.

While I have numerous problems with the conventional therapy for skin allergies, my greatest concern is that many doctors fail to give a proper diagnosis. Maybe these veterinarians don't want owners to have to spend much money in diagnosing their pets' problems. Maybe the doctors just decide that the pets have allergies, figure it's easy enough to treat them with corticosteroids or other medications that relieve the itchiness and red skin, and hope that the pet doesn't experience any serious side effects. This reasoning is no excuse for failing to diagnose and treat the pet correctly.

While skin allergies are certainly the most common cause of chronic itchiness in dogs, other more serious conditions can also cause dogs to scratch incessantly. These conditions include infections (bacterial or fungal such as ringworm), parasites (mange), immune disorders, *Malassezia* (yeast) dermatitis, contact dermatitis, skin cancers, and hormonal disorders such as hypothyroidism and Cushing's disease. Allergies other than atopic dermatitis can also be the problem; food allergies and flea allergy dermatitis are common culprits. These other causes are discussed at length in chapter 2.

> There is simply no excuse for failing to obtain a proper diagnosis prior to treatment of a chronic condition in a pet.

Only by performing diagnostic testing can a veterinarian find the real cause of the pet's chronic scratching and then treat the pet appropriately. There is simply no excuse for failing to obtain a proper diagnosis prior to treatment of a chronic condition in a pet. With a proper diagnosis, doctors are then in a position to refer those cases they are uncomfortable handling.

Another thing that is quite troubling to me is that so many pets with chronic allergies are being treated for months or years with potentially harmful medicines, usually steroids and antihistamines, without attempting other safer therapies. The lack of safe, long-term, and effective conventional treatments for allergic pets is the reason I first became interested in complementary therapies. I was frustrated at seeing the same pets in my hospital month after month for their "allergy" shot and dose of steroid pills. While I could help these pets stop itching for a few weeks, they would always come back for more drugs. I desperately wanted something to decrease their reliance on corticosteroids, which I knew could shorten their lives and was the cause of their side effects of increased appetite, increased intake of food and water, increased urination, and weight gain.

By getting "turned on" to the many complementary therapies available to help pets, I was able to finally offer my patients something other than only conventional medicines that temporarily covered up their symptoms without really addressing the problem and helping the pets heal.

## WHEN ALLERGIES DEVELOP

ATOPIC DERMATITIS IS a genetic disease, which makes some dogs predisposed to skin allergies. For this reason, dogs with atopy should not be bred. Due to the genetic component of the disease, certain breeds of dogs have a

# HOW ALLERGIES DEVELOP

The clinical signs of itching and inflammation seen in allergic pets occur as antibodies (proteins formed by the dog's white blood cells in response to contacting an allergen) contact environmental allergens and release their pro-inflammatory chemicals. Allergic dogs develop allergen-specific IgE antibodies and, to some extent, IgG antibodies. IgE antibodies are involved in Type I hypersensitivity reactions, the most common type of allergic reaction in the pet's body. The actual immunology is quite complicated.

IgE antibodies are formed upon exposure to an environmental allergen such as mold, human dander, fleas, house dust mites, or pollen from grasses, weeds, and trees. The IgE antibody attaches to a tissue cell called a mast cell. The next time the pet encounters the allergen, the allergen attaches to the IgE antibody-mast cell combination. Upon attachment to the IgE-mast cell unit, the mast cell disintegrates or "explodes," releasing the many chemicals contained within the cell and cell membrane. Some of these chemicals include histamine, substance P, bradykinin, and various prostaglandins. It is the presence of these chemicals that causes the clinical signs including inflammation and itching seen in allergic pets.

high incidence of atopic dermatitis. These breeds include Cairn Terriers, Shar-peis, West Highland White Terriers, Scottish Terriers, Lhasa Apsos, Shih Tzus, Wirehaired Fox Terriers, Dalmatians, Pugs, Irish Setters, Boston Terriers, Golden Retrievers, Boxers, English Setters, Labrador Retrievers, Miniature Schnauzers, and Belgian Tervurens. Some (but not all) studies show that females are affected more than males. Despite breed predisposition, atopic dermatitis can occur in any breed of dog.

According to the veterinary medicine literature, allergies usually show up in pets at 1 to 3 years of age. This is a bit misleading. Actually, allergies usually occur within 1 to 3 years of a pet being exposed to continual environmental allergens. If you live in an environment where there are few environmental allergens, even if your dog has the genetic predisposition to develop allergies, he will likely not do so. If you move to another area where there are many environmental allergens, such as here in Texas where I live, your genetically predisposed allergic dog will probably develop signs of allergies within 1 to 3 years of moving into the new environment.

Despite this well-reported figure of 1 to 3 years of age, or more correctly 1 to 3 years of ongoing antigen exposure, some pets do not show signs of allergies until midlife or later. Still others show signs from as early as a few months of age, barely into their puppyhood. While we can use age as a rough guideline, this is not a strict rule for pets with allergies.

When owners ask if allergies in their pets can be cured, the answer is usually no, although the rare pet "outgrows" his allergies. If an owner were to move to another place where there are few allergens that affect the dog, however, the allergic dog, while still technically "allergic," may not show signs of allergies and appear "cured."

# SIGNS OF ALLERGIES

ITCHING IS THE most obvious sign of atopic dermatitis. While skin lesions and discoloring of the skin are not a symptom of the disease itself, the constant self-trauma of scratching can cause skin lesions that lead to other problems, including secondary bacterial or yeast infections. Some dogs develop additional problems from the atopic disease, such as chronic ear infections, runny nose, and diarrhea.

Many atopic pets have only seasonal signs, showing itching during the season when the specific allergens to which they are allergic are most prominent. For example, pets with allergies to Bermuda grass living in my area of Texas often begin showing allergic signs in the spring when the grass begins to awaken after the winter. Eventually, however, most allergic pets develop signs that last all year long.

You can suspect atopic dermatitis if your dog itches, but his skin appears normal. (One exception mentioned in a leading dermatology text is that the English bulldog may have red skin with minimal itching.) This helps differentiate allergic atopy from other diseases that cause itchiness, but also produce skin lesions. The itchiness can be mild, moderate, or severe, but most allergic pets do not start off with severe itching. For a pet with sudden severe itching, I am more likely to suspect mange, fleas, or the rarely seen food allergies as the diagnosis.

With time, skin lesions and secondary infections can occur as a result of chronic scratching. Many dogs with chronic allergies develop pink or red skin, and bronzing and darkening of the skin. The pink or red color, which can also be seen early in the course of the disease, is from chronic inflammation. The bronzing effect is from pigment in the dog's saliva that discolors the skin and hair. This bronzing, which can also be seen early in the condition in dogs that excessively lick, is particularly striking in light-haired dogs. Darkening of the skin, called hyperpigmentation, can develop in any chronic skin disorder as the result of repeated trauma and inflammation.

Many dogs with atopic dermatitis also have flea allergies and chronic bacterial infections. Chronic skin infections are so common in allergic dogs that every dog with chronic skin infections should be screened for atopy and also for hormonal diseases such as hypothyroidism, another overlooked underlying disorder. Since allergic skin is not normal skin, it is predisposed to secondary infections. Most commonly, staphylococcal bacteria infect the skin, causing small red bumps called papules or small, pimple-like lesions called pustules. Scabs can also form when the papules or pustules rupture.

> For a pet with sudden severe itching, I am more likely to suspect mange, fleas, or the rarely seen food allergies as the diagnosis.

Secondary yeast infections are becoming increasingly common in atopic dogs. Most of the time the yeast *Malassezia* is the culprit. Dogs with yeast infections are typically quite itchy, with greasy yellow scales, red, and quite smelly. Yeast infections are often misdiagnosed, but should be considered in any dog with these signs.

Some dogs with allergies have atypical (non-dermatological) signs associated with their allergies. These can include runny nose, runny eyes, asthma (wheezing,) vomiting, and diarrhea. While people with allergies typically have

## VACCINATING ATOPIC PETS

Any foreign protein, including those found in vaccines, can tip the delicate balance in your atopic pet and cause an outbreak of allergies that result in scratching. Use care when administering vaccines. I do not vaccinate pets during an allergy outbreak, preferring instead to get the pet's immune system back into balance so it can maintain the proper degree of health. When vaccines are needed, I prefer to rely on vaccine titers (blood tests which show a pet's antibody level to a specific disease) to tell me which vaccines might be needed. (A more thorough discussion of vaccine titers can be found in the *Natural Health Bible for Dogs & Cats*, Prima Publishing, due out early 2001.)

If I do administer vaccines, I increase the pet's nutritional supplements and often add others (especially whole-food supplements) to strengthen the liver, help detoxify the pet, and support its immune system. If your atopic pet has shown allergic vaccine reactions, it is probably best never to immunize again, although this is something to discuss with your pet's doctor.

the syndrome of runny eyes and runny nose, this sign is not common in pets with allergies. Over the last few years, however, my veterinary colleagues and I have seen an increasing (though still small) number of dogs with sneezing and the runny eyes/runny nose syndrome that responds to conventional therapy for allergies. These dogs could be incorrectly treated with antibiotics for upper respiratory infections; owners should be aware that pets with these symptoms may in fact have mild allergic rhinitis—allergies causing a runny nose with a clear discharge.

Sadly, chronic ear and skin infections are common in atopic pets. Some dogs with chronic allergies—both atopic dermatitis and, rarely, true food allergies—only show chronic ear infections as their allergy symptom. Recurring skin and ear infections are not normal for dogs. If your dog has these chronic disorders, suspect that it has an underlying immune problem such as atopic dermatitis, food allergy, or thyroid or adrenal gland disease.

> While people with allergies typically have the syndrome of runny eyes and runny nose, this sign is not common in pets with allergies.

## FROM MY PATIENT FILES

WOLFIE WAS ONE of my first patients whose symptoms I suspected stemmed from a yeast infection with an underlying allergy problem. Wolfie is a 3-year-old Pekingese dog with a wonderful personality. When I first saw him, he was almost totally bald, had greasy skin, and emitted a horrible odor. He was quite a site to behold.

Wolfie's owner was desperate for help. Her prior veterinarian had diagnosed allergies and treated Wolfie with monthly injections of long-acting and potent steroids. Over time, Wolfie began to lose his hair and develop his greasy, smelly skin condition. The previous veterinarian then added insult to injury by adding potent antibiotics to the steroid regimen to treat what he termed a "skin infection."

Since the previous doctor had not tested Wolfie's skin disorder, I performed a skin scraping to check for mange, skin cytology (a microscopic examination of the skin cells obtained on a cotton swab rolled onto the skin) to check for yeasts and bacteria, and a blood profile specifically looking for evidence of thyroid disease. The skin scraping and blood profile were normal. The skin cytology did show the presence of a very small number of yeast *(Malassezia)* organisms. This secondary yeast infection was most likely due to the chronic use of corticosteroids and antibiotics and a failure to properly treat the underlying allergic dermatitis.

I knew that Wolfie would be a tough case due to his chronic history and horrible-looking skin. I treated him with medicated shampoos, followed by vinegar and water rinses to help resolve the yeast infection, a change of diet to a more natural food, and a number of nutritional supplements. Many doctors use potentially toxic drugs like ketoconazole to help treat *Malassezia* infections, but most of my patients respond to an aggressive regimen of nutritional supplements and very frequent—even daily at first—bathing and rinsing with the vinegar-and-water mix. A recheck in one month showed much improvement. Wolfie continues to do well to this day despite the occasional need for corticosteroids when he suffers a relapse of his allergies.

Genie is a sweet 5-year-old female Golden Retriever whose owner sought my assistance after conventional medicine failed to help her dog. It seems that Genie had been having problems with recurring ear infections for over 2 years. Upon questioning the owner, I was not surprised to learn that Genie had been treated with a number of conventional ear medicines over that time. The typical history is that the prescribed medication works while being administered but, within a few weeks of stopping the treatment, the ears become infected again. This was the case with Genie.

Genie's owner told me something else that did not surprise me: no diagnostic testing had been done to determine the cause of her infections. In order to treat an ear infection properly, it is necessary to determine the cause. Most of the ear infections I have seen in my years of practice were caused by the yeast *Malassezia;* I have diagnosed only a few cases of bacterial ear infection. While most pet owners tend to suspect ear mites as the cause of a pet's ear problems, mites are actually only rarely diagnosed, except in puppies, kittens, and stray pets.

A simple ear swab and a look under the microscope at the "goop" I extracted from Genie's inflamed ear canals revealed the *Malassezia* yeast organisms. Since her ears were tender and inflamed, I sedated Genie in order to perform a thorough ear cleaning and get a better look inside the ear canals. Genie's owner stated that her dog had never had her ears thoroughly cleaned at her previous doctor's office. Failing to properly clean the ears, which often requires sedation in dogs with painful ears, like Genie, is a major reason that treatment fails. After all, whatever medicine is used can't possibly make its way through an ear full of pus!

> Although atopic allergies are the most common cause of itchiness in dogs, there can be other causes.

The cleaning and otoscopic examination of Genie's ear canals went well. I detected no foreign bodies or tumors in her ears. Given Genie's history of chronic ear infections, I suspected an underlying cause. Since the thyroid test I ran came back normal, I suspected atopic dermatitis with a possible contribution by a dietary sensitivity to the "premium" diet Genie was fed. Her food contained animal by-products and chemical preservatives, which I knew did not make for the healthiest diet.

I treated Genie with the proper antifungal medication for *Malassezia,* then prescribed a regular regimen of ear cleaning with an herbal product I often use. I also changed her diet to a natural processed food because Genie's owner was unable to prepare food at home for her, and placed her on a variety of natural supplements I commonly use for treating allergies in pets.

To date, Genie is doing quite well, with only an occasional flare-up of ear infections. Her owner is quite pleased with her progress. While the staff and I love to see Genie when she comes to visit, her owner is glad that our proper diagnosis and natural treatment regimen have reduced her number of veterinary visits and lowered the cost of Genie's health care!

From the cases of Wolfie and Genie, you can see how obtaining a proper diagnosis of your pet's condition can mean the difference between illness and health. Although atopic dermatitis is the most common cause of itchiness in dogs, there can be other causes. It is very important that you get a diagnosis of your dog's problem as soon as possible so you and your veterinarian can take action to lessen the effect of the allergy before secondary infections occur. Or if something else is causing the problem, you can discover and solve whatever that is before the condition gets worse. Other causes of a dog scratching are discussed in the next chapter.

# CHAPTER SUMMARY

- Atopic dermatitis, commonly called skin allergies, is the most common cause of itchiness in dogs.

- Atopic dermatitis is a genetic disease.

- Genetics predispose a dog to react to environmental stimuli called allergens, such as dust mites and certain plant pollens.

- After the dog is exposed to the allergen for 1 to 3 years, the dog develops the allergic signs.

- The most common sign of allergies in a dog is scratching, often followed by secondary skin infections.

- Less common non-skin signs of atopic allergies include ear infections, runny nose, wheezing, vomiting, and diarrhea.

- Before beginning any treatment for your pet, be sure to receive a proper diagnosis.

# ·2·

# Not Allergies, But Something Else

MOST OF THE time the itch that compels a dog to scratch is caused by atopic dermatitis. A number of other skin problems that cause a dog to scratch are misdiagnosed as allergies, however. For this reason, I continually stress the importance of obtaining a proper diagnosis before embarking on therapy for a chronic condition in pets suspected of having allergies.

Rosie was a 4-year-old spayed female Rottweiler whose owners were a sweet couple who also had another pet, Baby, an 8-year-old female Miniature Poodle. When I first saw Rosie, she had just begun to scratch. Her skin looked normal, which told me she probably was not suffering from any parasite problems (such as fleas, ticks, or mange), bacterial infections (such as staphylococcal pyoderma), or the fungal infection ringworm. Baby was normal, neither scratching nor showing any skin lesions.

Neither of the dogs' owners had itchiness or skin problems. I always try to remember to ask owners about their own medical history because diseases such as sarcoptic mange and ringworm can be transmitted from pets to their owners and vice versa. A history of skin disease in the owners can help me in my efforts to diagnose the cause of the dermatitis in pets.

Due to her scratching and a negative skin scraping, despite normal skin, I tentatively diagnosed atopic dermatitis. Her owners decided to try a trial low dose of a corticosteroid called prednisolone rather than complementary therapies at that point.

At her recheck one week later, Rosie still looked normal but was scratching even more. A second skin scraping was also negative. I increased her dose of corticosteroids and also prescribed antihistamines for Rosie, with instructions to the owners to recheck her in another 1 to 2 weeks.

Once again, her recheck showed her scratching to be worse despite normal appearing skin. At this point, we elected to continue her medications but try a different antihistamine. I also prescribed an omega-3 fatty acid supplement, aloe vera-colloidal oatmeal shampoo and conditioner, and a hypoallergenic diet.

Ten days later, Rosie's scratching had increased and she now showed abrasions on her skin where she had scratched at herself. Once again, I repeated my examination and skin scraping (once again negative) and questioning of the owner. This time the owner mentioned that she and her husband had a few tiny itchy red bumps on the skin around their waistlines. I now knew the cause of Rosie's itching: sarcoptic mange!

While sarcoptic mange normally causes obvious skin lesions in dogs, in Rosie's case, she was afflicted with what has been called occult sarcoptic mange. In this disorder, the mange mites are in the dog's skin, but there is no clinical sign except itching. Skin scrapings are negative, as were all of Rosie's scrapings, and the itching gets worse, even with corticosteroid administration.

In this case, our trial dose of steroid should have relieved Rosie's itching if she suffered only from allergic (atopic) dermatitis. Her failure to respond to increasing doses of prednisolone told me that something other than allergies was causing her intense itching. When her owner showed me the tiny lesions she had developed on her body, these lesions plus Rosie's failure to respond to the corticosteroids told me what was wrong with her. This is a great example of a pet who had all the appearances of being allergic, but yet had another disorder that caused her to itch quite severely.

Mange is just one of several conditions misdiagnosed as allergic (atopic) dermatitis. Others range from ringworm and hormonal diseases to cancer and even behavioral problems. The following sections describe these conditions and their treatment options. Each can be treated by conventional and complementary therapies. Often a combination of the two used in a holistic approach is the best treatment. Any medication, and even some homeopathic remedies, can affect diagnostic tests and some drugs can cause a dermatitis reaction in some dogs. For these reasons, it is important to tell your veterinarian about all of the medicines, including heartworm and flea prevention medicines, that you give to your pet.

# MANGE

MANGE IS THE second most common cause (after atopic dermatitis) of scratching in dogs. A microscopic parasite called a mite infects the skin and hair follicles, resulting in

# CONDITIONS OFTEN MISDIAGNOSED AS ALLERGIC DERMATITIS

Demodectic mange
Sarcoptic mange
Fleabite hypersensitivity
Other insect hypersensitivity
Bacterial infection
*Malassezia* (yeast) dermatitis
Ringworm
Intestinal parasite hypersensitivity
Food allergies
Contact dermatitis
Drug reactions
Skin cancer
Thyroid and other hormonal diseases (hypothyroidism,
     Cushing's disease)
Behavioral problems (psychodermatosis)

mange. The two most common types of mange are demodectic mange and sarcoptic mange.

## Demodectic Mange
Demodectic mange is a genetic disease that can affect any dog, but most commonly strikes puppies under 12 months

# A CLOSER LOOK

Demodectic mange is commonly misdiagnosed in puppies and dogs. Most pets with demodectic mange are puppies with the mite-specific immune disorder. Due to a stronger immune system, older dogs rarely develop demodectic mange. Therefore, when an older dog develops demodectic mange, we must look for an underlying cause. In many cases, that cause is a serious condition affecting the immune system, such as cancer or endocrine disease (as in Cushing's disease). Older dogs taking high doses of corticosteroids for extended periods of time may also develop demodectic mange since corticosteroids suppress the immune system.

Older dogs with demodectic mange must be screened for underlying disorders of the immune system. Pet owners should keep in mind that in some pets, despite searching for an underlying immune system disorder, no underlying problems are found. These dogs must be closely monitored with veterinary visits and laboratory evaluation every 2 to 3 months to determine if a serious disorder arises.

of age. This type of mange is not transmissible to other pets or pet owners. Demodectic mange is caused by the mite *Demodex canis,* which is a normal inhabitant of the hair follicles of all dogs. The mites are transmitted by the mother dog to the puppies shortly after birth. Since all dogs carry demodectic mites in their hair follicles, yet only a few puppies or dogs ever develop the disease demodectic mange, obviously something has happened that allows these normal skin inhabitants to cause disease in the affected pets.

That something is a deficient immune system. Puppies that develop demodectic mange do not have a deficient immune system that predisposes them to every disease, however, only demodectic mange. Researchers now believe that the puppy that develops demodectic mange has a specific immune system defect, a mite-specific immunocompetence of varying severity, that allows the mites, normally living quietly in the hair follicles, to reproduce and cause disease.

There are two types of demodectic mange: localized mange or generalized mange. Localized mange causes one or more lesions on the body. Generalized mange causes lesions all over the body or all over a specific body area such as the feet and face. While localized mange is a mild disease, generalized mange is a very serious and potentially life-threatening condition. In the past, many dogs were euthanized due to the severe nature of the disorder, but now they can be treated.

> While localized mange is a mild disease, generalized mange is a very serious and potentially life-threatening condition.

Suspect local demodectic mange if the lesion is a patch—often a circular area—of hair loss that is pink or red and/or scaling. The pet is usually not itchy. Any body areas can be affected, but the most common areas in young puppies are the face and the forelegs. Most cases resolve within 1 to 2 months with topical treatment.

If the dog's entire body is affected, suspect generalized demodectic mange. (However, remember that this condition may involve only body regions such as the feet or face.) Areas of hair loss with red bumps called papules develop. If not diagnosed at this early stage, secondary infections often result, causing pimples or pustules with secondary seborrhea (dry or oily, flaky skin.) At this stage, strong antibiotics must be used to destroy the secondary infection.

With proper treatment, demodectic mange is curable in most dogs. In dogs that have been treated for the generalized form, corticosteroids should never be used except as a life-saving procedure, as the steroids can cause a relapse of the disease that can be difficult to treat.

Demodectic mange is often misdiagnosed in puppies and dogs. Since the disease can look like any skin disorder, all skin lesions that occur in puppies—and most if not all that occur in adult dogs—should be tested for mange. Testing is easy, involving a simple skin scraping made with a scalpel blade. (I prefer to use the edge of a glass slide to decrease the chance of cutting the pet or myself!)

The material from the skin scraping is placed on a drop of microscope oil on a slide, and examined for the mites. With very rare exception, if the pet has demodectic mange, the test will always show the mites, giving a positive result. The skin scraping must be a deep scraping since the mites live in the hair follicles. In sarcoptic mange, discussed below, a superficial skin scraping is adequate since the mites live in the superficial epidermal layer of skin. This is an important point because an incorrectly performed skin scraping will give an invalid result!

As demodectic mange is a genetic disease, affected dogs should be spayed or neutered and not bred. The parents of affected dogs should not be bred again.

## Sarcoptic Mange

The second type of mange commonly seen in dogs is called sarcoptic mange, also known as scabies. Sarcoptic mange is a very itchy disease and often misdiagnosed as allergies. Unlike demodectic mange, sarcoptic mange (caused by the mite *Sarcoptes scabiei* var canis) is easily transmitted to other pets in the household. This type of mange is also a zoonotic disease, meaning it can be transmitted to owners as well. In people who contract the disease from the family dog, skin lesions, usually small red itchy bumps called papules, occur within 24 hours of exposure. The mites live in the superficial layers of the skin and cause intense itching in affected pets. The itching can result from the presence of the mites themselves as they burrow into the skin, or from an allergic reaction to the mites.

Suspect sarcoptic mange if there are skin lesions on your dog's chest, abdomen, and legs, although they can occur anywhere on the body. The ears, ankles, and elbows are often involved. The lesions begin as papules that humans who contract the disease also get. The papules easily become irritated as the animal scratches, forming crusted lesions. While these classic lesions are seen in most dogs infected with sarcoptic mange mites, some dogs never develop these lesions or only develop them much later in the course of the disease, despite intense itching—like Rosie in the case at the beginning of the chapter. These dogs have occult sarcoptic mange.

Occult sarcoptic mange is easily confused with atopic dermatitis or food allergies. Despite ever increasing doses of corticosteroids, itching continues and gets worse. This failure to respond to what normally would be the proper dose of corticosteroids to resolve the itching of allergic dermatitis should prompt the doctor to suspect another cause, such as occult sarcoptic mange.

As with demodectic mange, skin scraping is the test most commonly used to diagnose sarcoptic mange. Although only a superficial skin scraping is needed to reveal the presence of the sarcoptic mange mites, I always perform a deep scraping as I never know which form of mange might be causing the clinical signs.

With demodectic mange, a deep skin scraping easily reveals the mites in almost 100 percent of affected dogs. Unfortunately, testing is not as dependable for sarcoptic mange. Multiple skin scrapings in dogs with sarcoptic mange only reveal the mites in approximately 50 percent of cases. The best place to take a scraping is from areas that have papules with crusts because they are most likely to reveal mites. Since the mites prefer the ear margins, elbows, and ankles of the dog, these sites should always be scraped for the testing.

Given that around 50 percent of affected dogs have negative skin scrapings, it is best to suspect the disease if your dog's severe itching does not respond to the typical "anti-itching" dose of corticosteroids. You should then treat your dog for sarcoptic mange. Since the disease is easily transmissible to other family pets, you need to treat all other pets in the household as well.

## Treatment Approaches for Mange

Conventional therapy for generalized demodectic mange involves dipping the pet every 1 to 2 weeks with a dip called Mitaban (amitraz). While a potent insecticide, side effects are rare, but can include vomiting, bloating, lethargy, and an

# A CLOSER LOOK

Pets with sarcoptic mange will improve with Mitaban dips or lime sulfur dips. Ivermectin, given as injections or oral medication, is more commonly used for this disorder, as it is considered less toxic than dipping. Do not treat collie-type dogs with ivermectin, as they may show toxic or fatal reactions with this drug. Corticosteroids can temporarily control the severe itching of dogs with sarcoptic mange, but do NOT use corticosteroids for pets with demodectic mange. It will worsen their condition.

unsteady gait. When your dog looks improved and has shown at least 1 or 2 negative skin scrapings, he is dipped twice more. At that point, the dipping treatment is complete. This often correlates to a series of 8 to 12 dips at a cost of $20 to $40 per dip.

Treatment for localized demodectic mange is the application of a topical ointment such as benzoyl peroxide to reduce inflammation. With topical treatment, some lesions temporarily look worse before they look better.

Complementary therapies for demodectic or sarcoptic mange include homeopathic remedies such as *Sulphur,* or herbal remedies such as echinacea or lavender, applied topically and/or given orally, depending upon the herb. I also recommend additional zinc and antioxidant vitamins and minerals to strengthen the immune system. You also might try giving your dog herbs containing natural plant steroids if he has sarcoptic mange. These herbs include ganoderma, ginseng, rehmannia, licorice, bupleurum, scute, *zizyphi fructus* (jujube), and sophora. Plant steroids usually have milder actions with minimal side effects compared to synthetic steroidal drugs. If the herbs are ineffective in controlling itching, you can try low doses of corticosteroids on a short-term basis, but only for dogs with sarcoptic mange. Corticosteroids will make demodectic mange worse.

Since demodectic mange can be quite devastating, any dog not responding to a short course of complementary therapy should receive the dips. Continue the complementary therapies to strengthen your dog's immune system and reduce the chances of side effects from the dipping.

> Corticosteroids will make demodectic mange worse.

## FLEABITE HYPERSENSITIVITY

FLEABITE HYPERSENSITIVITY, ALSO referred to as flea allergy dermatitis, is a common cause of itchy skin disease in dogs in many parts of the country. I used to diagnose this problem in most of my itchy patients. With the advent of the newer chemical flea control products that most conventional clients now use, the incidence of flea allergy cases has substantially decreased.

Suspect fleabite hypersensitivity if you see lesions mostly confined to the lower back, back and inner aspects of the thighs, abdomen, and flank areas. The typical lesions of flea allergy dermatitis are small red bumps (papules) that may be crusted. Since the location of these lesions are quite typical of flea allergy dermatitis and almost never occur with any other disease, you should consider a diagnosis of flea allergy dermatitis at the top of the list of possibilities until proven otherwise.

Owners often seem to dislike the diagnosis of flea allergy dermatitis, denying that the affected pet even has fleas. They may bathe itchy pets that have skin lesions to make them more comfortable. Bathing the pet removes any evidence of fleas, however, so I discourage owners coming to me for a second opinion from bathing their pets. Due to the immunology of flea allergy dermatitis, itchiness will persist long after the fleas have been removed from the pet. Many owners are doing some flea control (although it's not adequate if the dog has the condition), which decreases the chances that any fleas will be seen on the pet. Additionally, since flea allergy dermatitis can be quite itchy, it is not unusual to expect that the dog suffering from it will bite and kill the flea after the flea bites the dog! In other words, the dog himself removes any evidence of flea infestation.

> Suspect fleabite hypersensitivity if you see lesions mostly confined to the lower back, back and inner aspects of the thighs, abdomen, and flank areas.

Why do fleas bother some pets and not others? It is quite common in a multi-pet household for one pet to be allergic to fleas although not have any fleas while other pets do not seem bothered by fleas yet actually have fleas on them. In order to understand this phenomenon, it is important to understand the immunology behind this fascinating yet confusing skin disorder.

Flea saliva contains a number of antigenic (foreign protein) chemicals that are capable of inducing an allergic response in pets. In dogs, there are two types of immunologic reactions to flea saliva. The first is an immediate Type I hypersensitivity, similar to what occurs in atopic dermatitis. The pet feels itchy almost immediately after the flea bites. This is why he scratches, seeks out the flea, and kills it by chewing at it if he finds it.

There is also a delayed hypersensitivity response that may occur several days later, even though there may no longer be live fleas present. This is why many owners do not see fleas on the pet despite persistent and often quite severe itching.

Another interesting aspect of the immunology of flea allergy dermatitis involves the aspect of exposure. In the typical allergic situation, as with atopic dermatitis, exposure of the pet to the allergen causes the allergic reaction. Removing the offending allergens allows the pet to experience relief from the allergy.

> It is quite common in a multi-pet household for one pet to be allergic to fleas although not have any fleas while other pets do not seem bothered by fleas yet actually have fleas on them.

With flea allergy dermatitis, something unexpected occurs. Studies have shown that dogs continually exposed to fleas have low antibody levels and rarely develop allergic reactions to the fleas. Intermittent flea exposure, such as might occur with an indoor pet rarely exposed to fleas, induces both immediate and delayed allergic responses to flea saliva. Converting from intermittent to continuous exposure does not change these reactions. Many doctors have suggested that continuous exposure to fleas might in some way prevent flea allergy dermatitis.

Another interesting finding is that atopic dogs have a greater chance of developing a positive response to flea saliva. Thus, the atopic dog is also often allergic to fleas. This of course can confuse the diagnosis of an atopic dog that suddenly becomes infected with fleas. Careful evaluation is needed, and often both conditions require treatment.

History and physical examination are the bases of diagnosis. Ideally, fleas or flea excrement are found. Flea excrement is called flea "dirt," and resembles flecks of pepper on the pet's skin. You can easily test any black flecks seen on the pet to determine if they are flea excrement or simply scale from the pet. Place the black flecks on a white surface (towel, paper towel, white tabletop). Put a drop of water on each fleck. If the flecks are flea excrement, they will turn red within 30 to 60 seconds, whereas black scale will not. Since fleas eat blood when they feed on the pet, their droppings are dried blood, which the water rehydrates.

> Flea control is critical in controlling the ultimate cause of the pet's allergic dermatitis.

Finding flea dirt in the pet's feces is evidence of flea infestation. Also, since fleas carry tapeworms, finding tapeworm segments (called proglottid segments, which resemble small grains of rice) in the pet's feces is evidence of flea infestation.

As previously mentioned, you may not find fleas on pets with flea allergy dermatitis, but you usually find flea dirt. If owners have recently bathed the pet, of course, the presence of flea droppings is removed. Once again, it is important to point out that, ideally, you should not bathe your dog for 3 to 7 days prior to the office visit for the dermatology consult.

If the history and physical examination do not provide the diagnosis, your veterinarian can perform an intradermal skin test. A small amount of flea allergen is injected into the pet's skin and observed for a positive response.

A skin biopsy can also help determine the presence of flea allergy dermatitis. The test has limitations, however. It cannot definitely confirm the presence of flea allergy dermatitis, but rather only diagnoses allergic dermatitis. This is helpful in determining that the cause of the pet's dermatitis is an allergy (rather than something else, such as a fungal or bacterial infection or skin cancer), but further investigation is needed to determine the exact cause of the allergic dermatitis.

## Treatment Approaches for Fleabite Hypersensitivity

You can use conventional medications such as corticosteroids or antihistamines on a short-term basis to control the itching caused by insect bites. Complementary therapies that can control itching include the homeopathic remedies *Sulphur, Ledum,* or *Urtica urens,* and herbal remedies (echinacea, nettle, or lavender) applied topically and/or given orally, depending upon the herb. You also might try giving your dog herbs containing natural plant steroids. These herbs include ganoderma, ginseng, rehmannia, licorice, bupleurum, scute, *zizyphi fructus* (jujube), and sophora. Plant steroids usually have milder actions with minimal side effects compared to synthetic corticosteroids.

Flea control is critical in controlling the ultimate cause of the pet's allergic dermatitis. A thorough discussion of conventional versus complementary therapies for flea control is beyond the scope of this book. I refer the reader to the excellent and comprehensive discussion in the *Natural Health Bible for Dogs & Cats* (Prima Publishing, 2001).

Briefly, proper flea control must be directed at three sources: controlling fleas on the pet, in the yard, and in the house. Of the three, environmental flea control is the most important (and most neglected) as the majority of the flea life cycle is spent off the pet and in the environment. Conventional flea control involves insecticides: usually a pyrethrin-type chemical is applied in the house; an organophosphate-type chemical applied in the yard; and oral medicines such as Program or topical organophosphates such as Advantage or Front-Line applied on the pet.

> A holistic combination with short-term use of the safer of the conventional therapies and long-term maintenance with complementary therapies is the perfect flea control program.

Complementary therapies for flea control involve safer insecticides. Insect growth regulators, diatomaceous earth, or borate-type chemicals are used in the house. Beneficial nematodes and diatomaceous earth can be used in the yard. Neem shampoos and sprays, herbal collars, and powders can be applied on the pet for more natural topical flea control.

A holistic combination with short-term use of the safer of the conventional therapies and long-term maintenance with complementary therapies is the perfect flea control program.

# OTHER INSECT HYPERSENSITIVITY

MANY PET OWNERS suspect that insect bites are behind their dog's skin problems, often citing fire ants as the culprits. In reality, unlike people, it is the rare dog that develops problems related to other insect bites besides fleas.

Fire ants can and do bite dogs, but it is a rare occurrence. Ticks of course can attach themselves to dogs, but usually do not cause skin disease, although they do carry parasitic diseases such as Lyme disease, Rocky Mountain spotted fever, and ehrlichiosis. Flies can irritate dogs by biting the tips of the ears. Suspect this skin condition if you see oozing, crusted wounds on the tips and margins of the ears.

## Treatment Approaches for Insect Hypersensitivity

The conventional therapy is an antibiotic-corticosteroid ointment applied topically to the bites to help heal the wounds. For fly bites, topical insecticides are applied around the head to discourage the flies.

You can also try mange remedies for pets with itching caused by insect bites. Homeopathic remedies (such as *Sulphur, Ledum,* or *Urtica urens*) can help, as can herbal remedies (echinacea, nettle, or lavender) applied topically and/or given orally, depending upon the herb. You may want to try herbs containing natural plant steroids; these include ganoderma, ginseng, rehmannia, licorice, bupleurum, scute, zizyphi fructus (jujube), and sophora. The plant steroids usually have milder actions with minimal side effects compared to synthetic corticosteroids.

To hasten wound healing, apply topical herbal products that contain peppermint, chamomile, calendula, juniper, lavender, rose bark, or uva ursi. To prevent fly bites, try herbal products or products containing the insect repellent neem.

# Bacterial Infection

Skin problems caused by bacteria are a common diagnosis. The condition goes by a number of names, including bacterial folliculitis, pyoderma, or often simply "Staph infection." The cause is usually *Staphylococcus intermedius* (formerly improperly identified as *Staphylococcus aureus*), a bacterium that is normally present on the skin of dogs. Staphylococcal bacterial skin infections are usually related to an underlying cause such as allergies, parasitic infection, or a hormonal problem such as hypothyroidism or Cushing's disease. Undiagnosed and untreated demodectic mange routinely causes quite severe secondary bacterial infections.

In my experience, most chronically infected pets also have underlying allergic (atopic) dermatitis. Allergic skin is not "normal" skin and is more prone to infection. Allergic pets are particularly prone to secondary infections due to immune problems, damage to the skin from licking and chewing, which destroys the outer protective epidermal layer of skin, and chronic use of corticosteroids, especially long-acting injections.

Suspect bacterial infection if you see papules (small red bumps on the skin), pustules (pimples on the skin), and crusting. In shorthair dogs, a "moth-eaten" appearance to the coat is often the only sign.

Veterinarians usually diagnose bacterial infection based on visual inspection and ruling out other diseases of similar appearance, such as mange and ringworm. Skin biopsy can confirm diagnostic suspicions, but is usually not necessary.

Keep in mind with this diagnosis, however, that many pets, particularly those with chronic infections, have an underlying cause such as allergic dermatitis that must be addressed to prevent or decrease future bacterial infections.

Allergic skin is not "normal" skin and is more prone to infection.

## Treatment Approaches for Bacterial Infection

The conventional treatment for most bacterial infections is topical, injectable, or oral antibiotics. There are few good antibiotics that are effective in treating Staphylococcal dermatitis, and all are expensive. Proper antibiotic therapy should last at least 3 weeks or until 1 to 2 weeks beyond apparent cure. Topical medicated shampoos decrease itching, remove scales and crusts, decrease bacterial counts on the skin, and allow a shorter course of oral antibiotics or none at all for pets with mild infections treated at the first signs of infection. This is a great reason to see your veterinarian at the first signs of any illness, as early treatment may mean you can avoid resorting to conventional medications.

As to complementary therapies, once again I recommend the old standby homeopathic remedy, *Sulphur. Rhus toxicodendron, Silicea,* and *Hepar sulphuris* are also good. The homeopathic staphylococcus nosode is another option.

Herbal therapies include red clover, garlic, yellow dock, nettle, licorice root, echinacea, goldenseal, and German chamomile.

# MALASSEZIA DERMATITIS

THE YEAST *MALASSEZIA* is a newly recognized cause of skin problems in dogs. Under-diagnosed in pets, it is most often mistaken for simple atopic dermatitis or bacterial folliculitis.

The *Malassezia* yeast is commonly found in low numbers in ear canals and on the skin of the anal region and vagina of normal dogs. An alteration in the microenvironment of the skin allows the normally low numbers of yeasts to multiply and cause disease. Therefore, *Malassezia* dermatitis is usually considered a secondary rather than primary disease. First, the underlying atopic dermatitis, hypothyroidism, or Cushing's disease must be properly diagnosed and treated. Then the secondary yeast problem can be addressed.

Suspect *Malassezia* dermatitis if your dog is scratching at a moderate to severe degree. You may see inflammation of the skin, recognizable as increased pinkness or redness, along with excessive yellow scaling, greasiness, and a foul body odor. While the entire body can be affected, regional *Malassezia* dermatitis is also commonly diagnosed. The areas most typically involved are the ears, lips, underarms, elbows, neck, inner thighs, skin folds, anal area, and the area between the toes. *Malassezia* is the most common cause of ear disease in my practice; most pets with generalized *Malassezia* dermatitis also have *Malassezia* ear infections.

*Malassezia* dermatitis can afflict any breed. The breeds that seem most predisposed to it are Silky Terriers, Basset Hounds, Poodles, Shetland Sheepdogs, Collies, Chihuahuas, German Shepherds, Dachshunds, Australian Terriers, West

## A CLOSER LOOK

Three common fungi cause ringworm in pets: *Microsporum canis*, *Microsporum gypseum*, and *Trichophyton mentagrophytes*. *M. canis*, the most common cause, normally lives in small numbers in the skin and hair of dogs and cats. *M. gypseum* is a common fungus living in soil. Pets that become infected with this fungus normally acquire it after rooting in the dirt. *T. mentagrophytes* is commonly found on rodents; transmission typically requires contact with a rodent. Rarely, a dog develops ringworm after contact with an infected person harboring one of the fungi that can cause human ringworm. Most of the time, ringworm fungi are transmitted to pets through contact with infected animal hair or instruments such as combs and brushes that have contacted infected animal hair. While pets infected with ringworm can and do transmit ringworm to their owners, most people acquire ringworm from contact with an infected person or an infected person's brushes or combs.

Highland White Terriers, Jack Russell Terriers, Cocker Spaniels, and Springer Spaniels.

To diagnose the condition, veterinarians use a procedure called skin cytology to identify the *Malassezia* organisms on the skin. For this, a cotton swab is rolled over affected areas of skin and then gently rolled on a glass microscope slide. The slide is stained and then examined microscopically for the yeast organisms. Skin scrapings or skin tape preparations can also be used; some veterinarians consider these methods more reliable than skin cytology. Skin biopsy is usually not helpful in diagnosing this condition.

Given that an occasional yeast is a normal finding, most veterinary dermatologists believe that, in order to make a diagnosis of *Malassezia* dermatitis, a large number of organisms must be evident in skin cytology. I have made the diagnosis in many pets by finding only 1 or 2 *Malassezia* organisms, however. These patients exhibited the typical look and odor of patients with *Malassezia* dermatitis, suffered moderate to severe itching, had been treated with corticosteroids and/or antibiotics for months or years for "allergies" or "infections," and responded to treatment for *Malassezia* dermatitis. I use skin cytology as a guideline for diagnosing this condition, but treat for it if other signs point towards the diagnosis.

## Treatment Approaches for *Malassezia* Dermatitis

The conventional approach to treating *Malassezia* dermatitis is to wash the dog with medicated shampoos such as selenium sulfide, ketoconazole, zinc pyrithione, or chlorhexidine, followed by rinses of equal parts vinegar and water. Veterinarians also often prescribe oral ketoconazole, a potent antifungal drug. In my practice, I have had good success treating *Malassezia* dermatitis with aggressive topical therapy, without using the expensive and potentially toxic oral ketoconazole. If the latter is needed, a complete blood profile is necessary prior to starting treatment as the drug is toxic to the liver.

*Note:* When bathing a dog with medicated shampoo (or dipping a dog as mange treatment), wear protective gear such as goggles and gloves for safety.

I have not seen any recent reports of specific complementary therapies for the pet with *Malassezia* dermatitis. Any of the general therapies recommended for skin disorders are applicable, however. Frequent use of topical anti-yeast shampoos and the vinegar-water rinse can decrease the need for oral antifungal medications. Remember that yeast infections of the skin usually are secondary to some other condition that suppresses the immune system and allows the low concentrations of yeasts normally present on the skin to multiply out of control and cause disease. Once you discover the underlying immune problem, additional complementary therapies directed towards the problem are a good idea.

# Ringworm

Ringworm, called dermatophytosis in medical terms, is a common fungal infection in pets, specifically puppies and kittens. Long ago it was thought that a worm caused this disease, but it is now known that one of several fungi is actually the source. The condition was named after the appearance of the typical lesion, which is a circular or ring-shaped area of hair loss with crusting, especially around the periphery of the "ring."

Suspect ringworm if you see the classic circular area of hair loss, scale, and crusting. Ringworm can resemble any skin condition, however, and is often confused with bacterial folliculitis and mange. As a result, these three conditions must be suspected in any pet with any type of skin lesion. While infection with the soil fungus *M. gypseum* is rare, it causes a red raised nodule called a kerion on the face rather than the circular lesion typical of most ringworm infections. Usually, pets with ringworm are not itchy; if they are, it may suggest a parasitic or allergic problem as well.

Diagnosis is by visual inspection, ruling out other similar-looking problems, such as mange, by performing a skin scraping, and culturing hair and scale from the affected area. A crude test called a Wood's light test involves shining a fluorescent light on the affected area. Up to 50 percent of infections with the *M. canis* fungus will "glow in the dark." The test produces many false positive and false negative results, so should only be used as a screening test. Positive diagnosis requires performing a fungal culture.

> The rule of dermatology is: "If it looks like ringworm, it probably isn't; if it doesn't look like ringworm, it probably is ringworm."

The rule of dermatology is: "If it looks like ringworm, it probably isn't; if it doesn't look like ringworm, it probably is ringworm."

## Treatment Approaches for Ringworm

Treatment with conventional medications involves medicated shampoos and antifungal drugs (usually griseofulvin). Treatment is usually necessary for 4 to 6 weeks. In long-haired pets, clipping the hair will result in a greater chance for a cure.

Complementary therapies include improved nutrition. A more natural diet and supplementing with fatty acids and antioxidants are important. There is plenty of information about the role of diet in allergy prevention and general pet health in chapter 7. You might also try the homeopathic remedy *Sulphur,* and the herbs goldenseal and plantain.

# INTESTINAL PARASITE HYPERSENSITIVITY

INTESTINAL PARASITES ARE most commonly associated with gastrointestinal tract symptoms such as vomiting, diarrhea, blood in the feces, weight loss, a potbellied appearance, excess intestinal gas, intestinal cramping, and borborygmus (intestinal noise, that is, a noisy stomach), as well as anemia.

Intestinal parasites such as coccidia, roundworms, hookworms, tapeworms, and whipworms rarely cause a skin disorder. Doctors suspect that a Type I allergic hypersensitivity to parasites causes the itchiness in pets with this problem.

Suspect intestinal parasite hypersensitivity if your dog is scratching and has crusted papules and seborrhea. As with allergic dermatitis, sometimes the dog scratches, but has no skin lesions. Veterinarians use skin biopsy, positive fecal tests for intestinal parasites, and appropriate deworming to diagnose this condition.

## Treatment Approaches for Intestinal Parasite Hypersensitivity

Topical treatment involves shampooing the pet. Corticosteroids or complementary therapies for itching as discussed earlier can also be used as needed to give the pet relief. For a discussion of complementary therapies to control intestinal parasites, see the *Natural Health Bible for Dogs & Cats* (Prima Publishing, 2001).

# FOOD ALLERGIES

FOOD ALLERGIES OFTEN get the blame for a number of dermatological problems in dogs. In actuality, a true food allergy is quite rare, accounting for less than 10 percent of cases referred to veterinarians. Food allergies are far less common than atopic dermatitis. Food allergy or food hypersensitivity is a nonseasonal cause of severe itching in dogs, however.

Unlike the situation in most cases of allergic dermatitis, the itching in pets with food allergies is severe and intense and the itching most often does not respond to typical anti-inflammatory, anti-itching doses of corticosteroids.

Suspect food allergies when you have ruled out other causes. Food allergies can produce any number of lesions and, when the pet is suffering from severe itching, this hypersensitivity may be the cause. Secondary bacterial or yeast infections of the ears or skin can accompany food allergies, complicating the diagnosis.

About 10 to 15 percent of dogs with food allergies also have gastrointestinal problems such as vomiting, diarrhea, or abdominal discomfort (colic). Interestingly, some pets with seizures have food allergies; this is one of the many reasons why feeding a more natural diet is recommended for seizuring pets.

> Pets with food allergies may fare better if fed raw or minimally processed foods.

The hypersensitivity reaction occurs to one or more ingredients in the pet's food. In most cases, the pet has been eating the diet for months or years before the allergic reaction actually develops. Doctors suspect that most often a glycoprotein (a sugar-protein molecule) in the diet causes the allergic reaction. In many cases, cooking the food ingredient makes the pet's body recognize the glycoprotein as an allergen. Pets with food allergies may fare better if fed raw or minimally processed foods.

Food allergies can occur in any age or breed of dog. While the majority of cases are diagnosed in pets over two years of age, many dogs are less than 6 months old when they receive the diagnosis. There are several theories about why this may be so.

Younger pets commonly harbor intestinal parasites and viruses. It may be that these parasites or viruses in some way damage the intestinal mucosa, the inner lining of the intestine. Along with local antibodies, the mucosa serves as a protective layer to reduce the amount of foreign protein absorbed into the body. A damaged mucosa or defective antibody response allows food allergies to develop.

> Common food allergens include beef, chicken, milk, eggs, fish, wheat, soy, and corn, all of which are common ingredients in most pet foods.

In addition, very young animals eating commercial pet foods are exposed to a large number of antigenic substances. As the intestinal system is immature and has not adapted to these foreign substances, if this undigested material crosses the mucosa, an adverse food reaction may begin. The ability of any animal's immune system to "ignore" these foreign proteins is called oral tolerance. Without oral tolerance, pets—and people—would be allergic to anything entering the intestinal tract.

Tolerance develops at an early age. We are not sure of the exact age when a pet develops oral tolerance but at least one veterinarian, Dr. Donald Strombeck, believes it develops after 6 weeks of age, the typical age for weaning pets. Weaning at 8 to 10 weeks of age may be preferable. By the way, a later weaning is also preferable as a deterrent for behavioral problems that can develop later in life.

Common food allergens include beef, chicken, milk, eggs, fish, wheat, soy, and corn, all of which are common ingredients in most pet foods. Contrary to popular belief, lamb, like any other protein, is not hypoallergenic and can cause food allergies if fed over time. Most commercial foods contain large amounts of grain, an inexpensive source of energy for pets. These cereal grains contain large amounts of gluten, a carbohydrate that often causes pets to develop allergies. Delaying or preventing your dog from eating a diet with large amounts of cereal grains can allow oral tolerance to develop.

> Suspect food allergies if your dog has severe itching, especially nonseasonally, and it fails to respond to ever increasing doses of corticosteroids.

While there are no specific breeds that are predisposed to developing food allergies, some doctors feel that Cocker Spaniels, Springer Spaniels, Collies, Labrador Retrievers, Golden Retrievers, Miniature Schnauzers, Shar-peis, West Highland White Terriers, Boxers, Dalmatians, Dachshunds, Lhasa Apsos, German Shepherds, and Wheaton Terriers are at an increased risk.

Suspect food allergies if your dog has severe itching, especially nonseasonally, and it fails to respond to ever increasing doses of corticosteroids. Diagnosis is based on history, physical examination, and feeding an elimination or hypoallergenic diet. Blood testing, often conducted on pets with "allergies," is useless for diagnosing food allergies in pets. Simply switching from one commercial diet to another does not help pets with food allergies, as many brands contain similar ingredients. You need to work closely with your veterinarian to determine exactly what causes your dog's food reaction.

## The Elimination (Hypoallergenic) Diet

Feeding an elimination diet is the only way to accurately diagnose food allergies. After 8 to 12 weeks of eating the elimination diet, pets with food allergies have decreased itching or, in some cases, the itching is totally eliminated. The purpose of the elimination diet is to ban all protein that the dog has eaten before in order to isolate the allergen.

An elimination diet consists of 1 part protein and 4 to 5 parts cooked white rice. For dogs that have not eaten turkey or lamb, these are protein options. You can try any other protein sources that the dog has not eaten. If you are not sure of the protein sources he has had, try venison and rabbit, as few dogs have eaten these.

During the 8- to 12-week period, feed your pet only the prescribed diet. Absolutely no treats (including rawhide treats) or flavored heartworm preventive medication are allowed. As pets with food allergies are not allergic to drinking water, tap water can be offered. Many holistic-minded owners prefer bottled or distilled water; a recent study, however, showed that many brands of bottled water were no "purer" than tap water. During the food trial, avoid giving your pet any supplements, including vitamins and minerals. A healthy pet is unlikely to develop a nutritional deficiency in this short period of time.

Since up to 30 percent of pets with food allergies have other problems, including atopic dermatitis or flea

# LAMB AND RICE DIETS: WHAT YOU HAVEN'T BEEN TOLD

Recently, many pet owners have jumped on the "lamb and rice" bandwagon. While there is nothing inherently wrong with lamb and rice diets, the advertising developed to sell it can be misleading. Some pet food manufacturers have misled the average pet owner by claiming that lamb and rice diets are "hypoallergenic." In their attempts to sell yet another type of food, they have pushed lamb and rice diets as the newest, best things for pets.

Here are some things to consider before spending extra money on this special diet, which is not usually of any special benefit for your pet:

• While it is debated among doctors just how common food allergies really are, it is important to know that ANY food can cause food allergies. Many holistic practitioners believe that most commercial diets contribute to many illnesses, including food allergies and general ill health, whereas others believe that true food allergies are rare. As a cause of skin disease, food allergies are extremely rare in pets. Remember that less than 10 percent of puppies and dogs ever develop a true food allergy.

sensitivity, feeding the elimination diet may only reduce rather than solve the scratching problem completely. Here is one simple test to determine if food allergies are involved: If your dog returns to severe scratching when he returns to his regular diet, think food allergy.

• There is nothing inherently hypoallergenic about lamb or rice. Food allergies are more likely to be caused by a protein source that a pet has eaten for some period of time, often several years. Assuming your puppy is never exposed to lamb, he'll never develop an allergy to lamb. However, if you start feeding him a lamb-based diet, he can certainly become allergic to lamb later in life.

• Pets diagnosed with food allergies need a hypoallergenic diet. If your pet is used to eating lamb, it may be difficult and expensive to find a suitable diet. Other choices of protein for pets with food allergies include rabbit, fish, turkey, shrimp, lobster, or venison.

• Many lamb and rice diets also contain egg, wheat, soy, beef, fish, and chicken. Your dog could develop allergies to any or all of these substances despite eating a "lamb and rice" diet. If you choose to feed a lamb-based diet, read the label to see what else is in the food!

Since your pet doesn't derive any extra nutritional benefit from lamb, there is no particular reason to feed it to your dog although the diet won't hurt him if it is a natural diet.

If the itching decreases on the elimination diet, then add one ingredient at a time, checking to see if the itchiness returns, until you have developed a well-balanced diet that produces no itching reaction and so can be fed for the long term.

There are some pets who seem to do quite well when fed any homemade diet, yet develop problems, including itching, vomiting, and diarrhea, when fed a commercial diet. This is often the case even when the commercial diet contains similar ingredients as the homemade diet, such as the same protein and carbohydrate sources. The exact cause of this unusual situation is felt to be a food intolerance that develops to some additive, chemical, artificial coloring, preservative, or flavoring present in the commercial but not homemade diet. This is yet another reason why a natural, homemade diet is often preferable to a commercially prepared food.

While there are hypoallergenic prepared foods available by prescription from veterinarians, as of this writing there is no "natural" hypoallergenic pet food I can comfortably recommend for the elimination diet. Just like other commercial pet food, the commercially available hypoallergenic products may contain artificial and chemical preservatives and animal by-products. These ingredients throw off the test. Even the few natural diets not containing anything artificial, which are often recommended for "allergic" pets, usually have too many different ingredients to conduct a food trial properly. However, you can try these pet foods once it is determined which foreign proteins elicit allergic reactions, as long as the prepared food doesn't contain that type of protein.

For more information on diet and allergies, consult your holistic veterinarian. Also see chapter 7 for a discussion of natural feeding programs for pets with allergies.

Here are some concluding points concerning the diagnosis and treatment of food allergy dermatitis in pets, excerpted from a great handout called "Skin Disease, Food Allergy," written by two of the leading veterinary dermatologists, Dr. Lloyd Reedy and Dr. Reid Garfield.

# A CLOSER LOOK

Some medications that commonly cause drug reactions are:

Rabies vaccine (especially in Poodles and Terriers); sulfa drugs (especially in Doberman Pinschers and Miniature Schnauzers); various shampoos (in Miniature Schnauzers); daily heartworm preventative (cephalosporins, levamisole, cyclosporine, and diethylcarbamazine); penicillins; vaccines other than rabies vaccine; amitraz (the generic name of the dip Mitaban, used to treat demodectic mange); tetracycline; barbiturates; ivermectin (a commonly used dewormer and the ingredient in the monthly heartworm preventive Heartgard); various topical medications; and ear medications (Panalog and Tresaderm).

1. Food allergies cause nonseasonal dermatitis, itching, vomiting, diarrhea, and ear and skin infections.
2. Food allergies can begin at any age, but are most common in animals over 2 years of age.
3. Food allergies are much less common than atopic dermatitis.
4. Neither skin testing nor blood testing can accurately diagnose food allergy dermatitis. A feeding trial is necessary. Feeding trials require complete avoidance of everything except the recommended special diet.
5. Common allergens in food include beef, chicken, milk, eggs, fish, wheat, soy, and corn, all of which are common ingredients in most pet foods. Lamb is not

hypoallergenic and can cause food allergies if fed over time, like any other protein.

6. The test diet must be fed for up to 12 weeks, although some food allergic pets will respond before 12 weeks.

# CONTACT DERMATITIS

CONTACT DERMATITIS IS a rare cause of itching in pets. An inflammatory reaction caused by direct contact with the offending allergen, contact dermatitis typically afflicts skin (usually of the ears) that has been treated with a topical medication. The skin reaction occurs quite suddenly following contact. In addition to ear medications, other agents often incriminated in contact dermatitis are soaps, disinfectants, weed killer, insecticides, fertilizers, and flea collars.

Flea collars are quite commonly the cause. The collars produce a circular area of hair loss and inflammation or redness around the neck. Soaps and yard care products often cause dermatitis on the abdomen, groin, and armpits of the pet. Pets that lick the foreign substance may also develop lesions of the mouth.

Appearance and history of exposure are used to diagnose contact dermatitis.

## Treatment Approaches for Contact Dermatitis

Conventional therapy involves washing away the irritant. Soothing products such as aloe vera with colloidal oatmeal used as a spray or rinse, serve as complementary therapies to ease inflammation. Homeopathic remedies include *Sulphur, Ledum,* or *Urtica urens,* and herbal remedies (echinacea, nettle, or lavender) applied topically and/or given orally, depending upon the herb. You also might try giving your dog herbs containing natural plant steroids. These herbs include ganoderma, ginseng, rehmannia, licorice, bupleurum, scute, *zizyphi fructus* (jujube), and sophora. Plant steroids usually have milder actions with minimal side effects compared to synthetic corticosteroids. If these approaches are ineffective in controlling itching, you can try low doses of corticosteroids and antihistamines on a short-term basis, usually for less than 24 hours.

# DRUG REACTIONS

ADVERSE DRUG REACTIONS are quite common in people, and skin lesions often result as part of the reaction. In pets, reactions to medications are less common. They occur in approximately three out of every 1,000 patients, and do cause dogs to scratch. Any medication can be involved, and any route of administration (oral, topical, injection, or inhalation) can induce an allergic reaction.

Drug reactions can mimic any skin disease including atopic dermatitis. Most reactions occur within 1 to 2 weeks of administering the medication, but drug reactions can occur after a pet has been receiving the drug for days, or even years, or a few days after drug therapy is discontinued.

Any medication or complementary treatment can cause an allergic reaction. Some drug reactions are predictable. An example is a chemotherapy medication or immunosuppressive medicine that can cause hair loss or itching. Other drug

> Any medication or complementary treatment can cause an allergic reaction.

reactions are unpredictable, occurring as some result of the individual pet's immunologic response or genetic susceptibility.

Suspect a drug reaction based upon history and skin biopsy, and improvement after stopping the drug. Note that stopping use will not always help, as in the case of severe and potentially fatal drug reactions such as the reaction called toxic epidermal necrolysis.

# Behavioral Problems

EMOTIONAL RATHER THAN physical factors may be the reason some pets constantly scratch. An often-overlooked cause of scratching in pets is called psychodermatosis, behavioral stress that causes the dog to scratch. In these rare but challenging cases, some behavioral distress causes the pet to excessively lick or chew at his body. The lesions you see are a result of damage done by the pet to the skin and can include simply hair loss or raw, hot-spot-type lesions. In general, doctors believe that this disorder represents some sort of obsessive-compulsive disorder similar to that causing people to excessively chew their fingernails.

Causes of psychodermatosis are varied and difficult to pinpoint. Breed predisposition is one possibility. Nervous breeds such as Doberman Pinschers, Great Danes, Labrador Retrievers, Irish Setters, and German Shepherds often exhibit this behavior. Lifestyle issues, such as forced isolation away from the owner for breeds requiring a large amount of exercise and companionship, can cause psychodermatosis. A pet that is particularly nervous or bonded to his owner may begin scratching uncontrollably when separated from his human.

Based on history and the appearance of the lesion, diagnosis can be easy or quite difficult. A number of dermatological skin tests, including skin biopsy, may be indicated to make sure a more serious problem such as skin cancer is not involved.

### Treatment Approaches for Behavioral Problems

Conventional treatment involves behavior modifying medications and training. Complementary therapy includes behavior modification and behavior modifying herbs such as kava kava or flower essences such as Rescue Remedy. Regardless of the approach chosen, training the pet to alter his anxiety is an important part of therapy that is often neglected by owners and veterinarians. Behavior therapy takes a lot of time and patience on the part of the owner; full cure takes time and may never occur.

# SKIN CANCER

WHILE NOT USUALLY a cause of scratching in pets, skin cancers can produce a variety of lesions of the skin. Mast cell tumors, which contain histamine, can cause local itchiness. You should have any unusual lumps, bumps, or skin lesions on your pet examined by a veterinarian. Too many owners (and unfortunately, many doctors) fail to properly identify skin lesions, simply preferring to "guess" that they represent fatty tumors or cysts. *Benign, noncancerous skin lesions look just like cancerous skin lesions.* Therefore, veterinarians should aspirate or biopsy lumps and bumps rather than just "watch to see what happens." For the holistic-minded pet owner and doctor, watching a cancerous lump spread and ultimately kill the pet makes no sense. Skin warts, called papillomas, usually cause no problems and can be left alone or removed, at the owner's discretion.

# THYROID AND OTHER HORMONAL DISEASES

THYROID DISEASE IS under-diagnosed and is often the cause of a whole host of chronic diseases in dogs. Hypothyroidism, or low thyroid disease, is probably the most common hormonal (endocrine) disease that veterinarians diagnose in dogs. It is usually considered an autoimmune disease, in which the dog forms antibodies against his own thyroid gland. These antibodies result in the thyroid gland producing too little thyroid hormone.

When I was in veterinary school, we learned that the "classic signs" of hypothyroidism in dogs were obesity, hair loss, and the pet seeking warm places. Over the last few years, doctors have come to discover that thyroid dysfunction can have many clinical signs and resemble any number of diseases. Rarely do I see a pet with the "classic signs" of thyroid disease.

Not long ago, I encountered a very unusual case of hypothyroidism. I discussed this case in the book *The Arthritis Solution for Dogs* (Prima Publishing), since the patient had signs of both "arthritis" and "allergies" as a result of his thyroid condition.

Angus was originally referred to me for acupuncture for presumed hip dysplasia. For a more detailed discussion of how hypothyroidism can mimic signs of hip dysplasia and arthritis, I refer you to *The Arthritis Solution for Dogs*. For this discussion, I'll limit my comments to his misdiagnosis of "allergies."

Angus was a 7-year-old male neutered Rottweiler, whose owner brought him to me for a third opinion, to evaluate him for possible arthritis secondary to hip dysplasia. I estimated that Angus, at 149 pounds, was 30 to 40 pounds overweight. His owner confirmed that, reporting that his normal weight was 120 pounds. Recently, Angus had showed difficulty moving around. Beginning about 2 to 3 weeks prior to our visit, he had grown more lethargic. Within the last week prior to our visit, according to his owner, when he stood up from a prone position, he "staggered as if he was drunk."

Prior medical history provided by his owner revealed recurrent staphylococcal pyoderma, a common bacterial skin infection in dogs, that was responsive to various antibiotics. His original veterinarian had mentioned the possibility of allergic atopic dermatitis as a cause of Angus' constant scratching and recurring skin infections, but no testing was done to determine this. Angus' diet consisted of a premium obesity prevention diet, although he did not lose weight while eating this diet.

> Hypothyroidism, or low thyroid disease, is probably the most common hormonal (endocrine) disease that veterinarians diagnose in dogs.

Physical examination in my office showed an obese dog who was stiff and slow moving. I noted no pain upon manipulation of his limbs. I did note pelvic limb swaying, resembling a drunken swagger, but detected no neurological deficits in either the front or rear limbs. Cranial nerve functioning was within normal limits, indicating no problems or diseases of the brain. Angus seemed to have mild, nonpainful swelling of both front feet; no fever was detected.

Angus had no exposure to external parasites such as fleas and ticks, according to the owner.

When I listened to Angus' chest, I noticed no abnormal heart or lung sounds; his pulses were strong and regular. Abdominal and lymph node examination appeared to be normal. Peripheral lymph nodes were not enlarged. Grade II periodontal disease was detected based upon excessive tartar on his teeth. A voided urine sample was normal. A review of Angus' pelvic radiograph showed that they were underexposed, with a "froggy view" of the hip joints. The films were made without sedation and the correct ventrodorsal view, required to properly evaluate the hip joints, was not obtained. Despite these shortcomings, it was apparent that hip dysplasia and secondary arthritis were not the cause of Angus' clinical signs. As is typical of at least half of the cases that come to me for complementary therapies for "arthritis," Angus in fact had perfectly normal hips that did not require treatment.

What then was the cause of Angus' clinical signs that was misdiagnosed by the previous two doctors who examined Angus? Based on Angus' sudden onset of lethargy and swaggering gait, his lack of response to nonsteroidal medication to treat apparent hip dysplasia, and his history of recurring skin disease, I ordered a CBC and biochemical blood profile. The profile revealed high cholesterol, anemia, and very low thyroid hormone levels. The diagnosis was easy to make: Angus suffered from hypothyroidism, and this was the cause of all of his clinical signs and abnormal blood results.

After I prescribed thyroid supplements and a weight loss diet, Angus' signs and blood values returned to normal. To date, he is doing very well, walking normally, and is near his ideal weight. Additionally, because hypothyroidism can cause chronic skin infections, now that Angus' thyroid disease is under control Angus experiences fewer skin infections.

Angus may also have allergic (atopic) dermatitis, as pets with skin disease can have more than one underlying cause of their problems. This of course can confuse pet owners, complicate the diagnosis and treatment, and be quite frustrating for both the owner and the doctor. The answer will be revealed if signs of allergic dermatitis recur. For now, Angus' skin is much improved since I made the diagnosis of hypothyroidism and instituted proper treatment.

While Angus' case was quite unusual, it demonstrates that any number of disorders can cause signs that resemble allergies. Recurring skin infections should prompt a search for another disorder. It is imperative that proper diagnostic testing is performed in order to arrive at the correct diagnosis and offer the best treatment. Testing is discussed in the next chapter.

# CHAPTER SUMMARY

- It is very important to have your dog properly diagnosed before beginning treatment for allergies.

- Although atopic dermatitis is the most common cause of scratching in dogs, there are other causes.

- Mange is the second most common cause of scratching.

- Hypersensitivity to insects, fleas, drugs, allergen contact, or food content can cause skin problems.

- Skin lesions and scratching may also be a sign of skin cancer or thyroid disease.

- There are conventional treatments and complementary therapies for causes of scratching.

# ·3·

# What to Expect from Your Veterinarian

WHAT SHOULD YOU expect when you visit your veterinarian with a pet showing signs of skin allergies? The kind of care the dog will receive depends upon the veterinarian. A "100 percent conventional" doctor who is closed-minded toward complementary therapies has one approach, while a "100 percent alternative" doctor who is closed-minded toward conventional treatments offers a totally different experience.

Veterinarians who are 100 percent conventional don't even consider such therapies as acupuncture, herbal medicine, and nutritional supplements. Instead, they rely only on conventional medications. Some of these doctors don't offer much in the way of diagnostics, preferring instead to try various medications and take a "wait and see" approach.

Conversely, 100 percent alternative medicine veterinarians are not generally open to using conventional drugs for short-term itching and inflammation relief. These doctors may not use a lot of conventional diagnostic testing either, but for different reasons than the 100 percent conventional doctors. They prefer to use alternative diagnostic techniques and to treat your pet based upon clinical signs.

I believe the best doctor is one who is truly holistic, one who offers both conventional and alternative therapy approaches, and uses them to complement each other, just as I have tried to do in this book. By being open to doing whatever is in the animal's best interest, the veterinarian offers your pet the best care possible.

# Practicing Holistic Medicine

As I lecture to pet owners and give interviews to promote this series of health guides, I'm often asked why more doctors don't practice holistic medicine. I believe there are several answers to this question.

First, veterinarians really aren't trained to be holistic doctors. Few if any veterinary schools teach about wellness programs and disease prevention. Medical schools have just begun to introduce this information into their curriculums. I believe veterinary schools will eventually adapt to this philosophy, although it will take some time.

Traditional pharmacology courses in veterinary schools focus only on conventional drug therapies and ignore the more natural treatments such as herbal remedies. While it is vitally important to know about the many wonderful medications available, a few lectures on the more natural treatments would expose the doctors-to-be to these exciting therapies.

When I was in school, the focus was on diagnosis and treatment of diseases through recognition of signs and symptoms. While it certainly is important to diagnose and treat diseases, it's more important to prevent as many of these problems as possible, which is the holistic doctor's approach.

The second reason few doctors practice holistic medicine is that it takes time, and a lot of it. Standard veterinary practices book four or more appointments per hour. Since it takes longer to take a complete patient history and personalize a wellness disease prevention program for each patient, the holistic practice books just one to two appointments per hour.

The third reason there are few holistic veterinarians is fear. There are still a large number of doctors who believe that anything other than conventional medicine is quackish. I get a lot of mail from doctors upset that I propose any treatments that have not been subjected to a number of double-blind studies. While I too hope for the day when more of our complementary therapies can receive funding to undergo these rigorous trials, I must accept the clinical data we have now and do

> If your doctor is not open to a holistic approach, find one who is.

what I can to help my patients. While it is true that there are certainly some charlatans out there, and there are some complementary treatments of questionable value, by and large there is considerable evidence for the success of most mainstream complementary therapies. I don't think I need to run expensive tests to show, for example, that the approximately 4000-year-old practice of acupuncture has merit. This is one therapy that has stood the test of time.

## Finding a Holistic Veterinarian

You may have to do some research to find a really good doctor who has this much-needed holistic philosophy. Begin by evaluating your pet's current veterinarian. If he or she is open to complementary therapies, your current doctor can treat your pet's basic needs with a holistic approach, and refer you to a doctor who performs complementary therapies when those are needed. If your doctor is not open to a holistic approach, find one who is.

As an aside, most doctors, even those that do not offer services like acupuncture and herbal medicine, are using nutritional supplements as part of their therapy for allergies. This means your own doctor might be able to offer your arthritic pet some basic complementary therapy without the need for referral. Hopefully, this trend towards using supplements as part of the treatment of various conditions will continue.

If your dog does not have a current doctor, or you do not feel that your current doctor can treat your pet holistically, ask someone you know who uses a holistic veterinarian for a referral. You can also ask for a referral at the local health food store, pet store, or natural grocery store. These places often get requests for referrals. Pet and health food stores often have directories with advertisements for holistic doctors and holistic veterinarians. You might also consult your phone book for veterinarians advertising holistic care. Finally, contact the American Holistic Veterinary Medical Association. You can reach them at 410-569-0795 and ask for referrals to doctors in your area.

> Make sure the doctor is open-minded to a variety of conventional and complementary therapies, and places your pet's overall health first.

# ASK THE VETERINARIAN

Whether you meet your prospective holistic veterinarians in person or speak to them on the telephone, be prepared with questions to make the interview easier and more productive. Consider these sample questions to ask the doctor who might end up treating your pet for atopic dermatitis:

**Question:** How do you make a definitive diagnosis of atopic dermatitis?
**Ideal answer:** This is done using a combination of tests including skin scrapings, fungal culture, skin biopsy, and blood tests including tests for thyroid disease.

**Question:** What are your feelings about using drugs to control itching?
**Ideal answer:** Short-term use of corticosteroids or antihistamines is acceptable on an as-needed basis, and varies from case to case. Chronic use of these medications is limited to the very rare pet that does not respond to any other therapy. Pets on chronic medical therapies require monitoring of vital signs every 2 to 3 months, and laboratory tests to allow early detection of serious and potentially fatal side effects.

**Question:** What type of diet should my pet eat?
**Ideal answer:** I recommend the most natural prepared food or homemade diet possible.

**Question:** How do you treat chronic cases of allergies?
**Ideal answer:** I use supplements, herbs, homeopathy, and acupuncture, and prescribe conventional medications on a short-term, as-needed basis.

None of these methods of tracking down a good holistic doctor are foolproof, but they give you a starting point. Compile a list of as many names as possible from these sources, and then make an appointment to visit with each doctor on your list. Make sure you and the doctor get along, because your relationship with your pet's doctor is key to your pet's health. Make sure the doctor is open-minded to a variety of conventional and complementary therapies, and places your pet's overall health first.

# The Doctor Visit

Once you've found the perfect doctor for you and arrived for your appointment, it is important to understand what should happen during your visit. If this is your first visit, expect to spend anywhere from 30 to 60 minutes or more for the initial evaluation and diagnostic testing. The visit is divided into three parts: the medical history, examination, and laboratory evaluation.

## The Medical History
The history you provide is vital in helping your doctor properly assess your pet. It guides him in knowing what areas of the body to pay particular attention to during his examination, and helps him select only those laboratory tests needed to arrive at a proper diagnosis. It is not uncommon for clients to bring me pages of notes they have made at home, as well as notes and medical records from a prior doctor to aid me in my search for the correct diagnosis and treatment.

## What to Bring with You
In order to get the most from your holistic veterinary visit, you must be an active participant. Begin your partici-

pation before your dog's appointment by gathering the following:

- Verify the onset of your dog's scratching. Be prepared with an accurate estimate of how long your pet has been troubled. If the problem occurs only occasionally, keep notes about the circumstances, such as the time of year, if a particular plant is in bloom in your area, or if you have been traveling or visiting a new outdoor area.

- Provide all your dog's medical records or at least the names, addresses, and telephone numbers of all doctors your dog has visited. If you are visiting this doctor for a second opinion on a diagnosis, bring the results of any tests that have already been performed.

- Make notes of all treatments you have tried, both conventional and complementary, and any effect these treatments had on your dog.

- Be sure to make the doctor aware of any medications, including heartworm medications and over-the-counter flea and tick preventions, that your dog is taking. Always bring in any medicine containers, even if empty, so the doctor can assess the prescription. Many times I find that the wrong dosage or dosing interval was prescribed. This can account for the pet failing to improve.

- Know the ingredients and amounts of all food your dog eats.

- Track as much as possible your dog's bowel and urinary output and any other signs of your dog's general health.

- Make a list of any other medical concerns your dog suffers from, in addition to the scratching. Other problems may indicate a diagnosis other than atopic dermatitis in the itchy pet, or simply indicate additional medical problems in your pet, which is not uncommon.

- Check yourself and other animal and human members of the household for signs of skin lesions.

## The Examination

After asking about medical history and any other questions of importance, your doctor will commence with the physical examination. I like to break the physical down into two parts: the general physical examination and the skin examination.

The general physical allows me to properly examine the pet from head to toe. During this part, I pretty much ignore the primary complaint of itching and skin disease so that I can detect any other problems that might exist. Sometimes these other problems are related to the itchiness; sometimes they just exist coincidentally with the skin disorder.

By thoroughly checking the patient over, I am truly offering holistic care. For example, suppose that during my overall physical I discover that the dog, originally brought in for itchiness, has a heart murmur indicating heart disease, or a tumor on the body that might be cancer. These problems can't be ignored and might actually take priority over the original problem. Therefore, all of my patients brought in, even for something as "simple" as scratching, need and receive a full and thorough physical examination.

The second part of the examination involves evaluating the skin. This dermatological examination allows me to focus in on the primary problem mentioned by the owner. During this part, I observe the pet at rest to see if signs of itchiness, such as scratching, licking, chewing, and rubbing, occur in the examination room. Most dogs with mild itchiness do not shows these signs in the hospital, whereas pets with moderate to severe itchiness often scratch, rub, chew, or lick at various body parts while I'm talking with the owner.

After observing the pet at rest, I like to get "up close and personal." This involves looking at the skin, all of the skin, from every conceivable angle. I look the pet over from head to toe again, but this time focusing on the skin. By examining the whole body, I see both older healing lesions and any new ones. I can also determine the degree of inflammation and examine the skin for parasites. I also like to look at the general condition of the coat, as well as the specific areas of hair surrounding places of abnormal skin. I pay particular attention to those areas of the body most likely affected in pets with atopic dermatitis: the armpits, the abdomen, the feet, and the groin. In all pets with a history of scratching, I closely examine the ears, often red and inflamed and secondarily infected with yeasts or bacteria.

> Most dogs with mild itchiness do not shows these signs in the hospital, whereas pets with moderate to severe itchiness often scratch, rub, chew, or lick at various body parts while I'm talking with the owner.

Since it is critical that I see the skin "at its worst," I discourage owners from bathing the pet or cleaning the ears several days prior to our visit. I don't want owners washing away any skin lesions that can aid me in formulating a proper diagnosis. I know it is often hard for owners not to bathe a pet whose condition involves skin odor and skin lesions, but washing away evidence of the problem harms my investigation into determining the exact cause of the dog's problems.

The final part of the examination involves inspection of the skin with a magnifying glass. With the naked eye, it's easy to overlook tiny lesions; proper lighting and magnification is essential in performing a proper dermatological examination.

## The Laboratory Evaluation

A laboratory evaluation is critical in distinguishing subtle clues detected during the two-part physical examination. It is often the most neglected part of the evaluation of the scratching animal, as evidenced by the number of pets in my practice who have been treated for "allergies" with potentially harmful medications, but have never had any laboratory evaluation. Tests for allergic atopic dermatitis include skin testing, in vitro blood testing, and skin biopsy. In addition, tests should be performed to discover or rule out the other common skin disorders discussed in chapter 2.

Pets who show signs of having atopic dermatitis can be tested to confirm the suspicion. If you and your veterinarian decide that antigen therapy (injections of small amounts of the allergens in an attempt to "immunize" your pet against the allergens) is a good option for your pet, testing also provides information necessary for the preparation of the allergens for that therapy.

## Skin Testing

The gold standard of allergy testing is skin testing, called intradermal allergy testing. In this procedure, tiny amounts of allergens are injected in several spots into the superficial layer of skin on the patient. Most pets can be fully awake for the procedure; fractious animals may require sedation. At 15 minutes and again at 30 minutes after the injections, the doctor inspects the injection sites and grades them as positive or negative reactions. (Positive means an allergic reaction, negative means no reaction.) Each test includes an injection of sterile water, which serves as a negative control for comparison, as well as an injection of histamine, which serves as a positive control, for comparison.

> The gold standard of allergy testing is skin testing, called intradermal allergy testing.

While experienced doctorss can visually interpret the reactions at the injection sites, most doctor prefer a more objective assessment and actually measure the sites and compare them to the positive and negative control injection sites. Since performing and interpreting the test requires some skill, only a veterinary dermatologist or general practitioner with experience in intradermal skin testing should perform the test.

There is always the chance of false positive and false negative reactions, even with careful performance of the test by an experienced doctor. A false positive reaction means that the test gives a positive result (meaning the pet is allergic), but the positive result is inaccurate. A false negative means that the test mistakenly shows that the dog is not allergic to a substance. Among the potential problems that must be considered when performing intradermal skin testing for the diagnosis of atopic dermatitis in pets are the following: selection of antigens to test, using allergen mixes, and prior use of medications.

**Selection of Antigens**  Intradermal skin testing works best when the doctor includes local antigens, as these are most likely to elicit a positive reaction in a truly allergic pet. Since pets develop allergies to local foreign proteins they are most likely to encounter, these regional or local allergens must be included in the test. For example, in my area, Bermuda grass is a big problem in most allergic dogs. Failing to include Bermuda grass allergen in the test would result in a failure to diagnose and properly treat a common allergen in allergic dogs in Plano, Texas. Likewise, including allergens that dogs in Plano are unlikely to encounter would not be beneficial. If a dog is unlikely to contact a pollen from a plant that only grows in California, including it in an intradermal test for a dog living in Plano is unnecessary. Remembering to tell the doctor about any unusual plants your dog encounters will help the doctor determine the antigens to test.

**Using Allergen Mixes**  Testing a mix of allergens at once is a shortcut in blood testing for allergies. Rather than testing a single allergen such as Bermuda grass, for example, a mix of grasses can be combined for testing. The problem with this is that it fails to identify the specific allergen that might cause an allergic reaction in the pet. The goal of intradermal testing is not just to confirm the diagnosis, but also prepare a solution of antigens to be used as treatment for the pet. Testing a mix doesn't provide the information needed to treat the individual allergies. The intradermal treatment solution prepared by this method might not include allergens that should be included, and may include allergens that do not need to be included.

For example, let's suppose a grass mixture, rather than individual grasses, is used to test the dog with suspected allergic dermatitis. Let us further suppose this allergen mixture includes Bermuda grass, rye grass, timothy grass, and clover grass. Now assume that the dog is only allergic to Bermuda grass. The dog would show a positive reaction to Bermuda grass if it were tested by itself. Since Bermuda grass only makes up 25 percent of the grass mixture, testing the mix of grasses might yield a negative (a false negative) reaction since the dog is not allergic to 75 percent of the allergens in the mix. This means that Bermuda grass, to which the dog is highly allergic, would not be included in the antigen mix (made up of all the allergens that tested positive) used for treatment, dooming the owner to expensive long-term treatment that won't work.

Conversely, let's suppose that another dog is allergic to Bermuda and rye grass, but not allergic to timothy or clover. In testing the individual allergens, we would see a positive response to Bermuda and rye, but a negative response to timothy and clover. It is likely that testing a mix of these four potential allergens would produce a positive response in a dog allergic to two of the grasses. The final treatment mixture of antigens would contain all four grasses, yet the dog is not allergic to half of the grasses in the mix! The dog would be overtreated with antigens he does not need, which also might result in treatment failure at considerable expense to the owner and suffering of the patient.

Therefore, I strongly recommend testing individual antigens rather than mixes. It takes more time, but is much more accurate.

**Prior Use of Medications**    False negative reactions commonly occur if the pet has recently been treated with the following medications: corticosteroids, antihistamines, and progesterone compounds. Supplementing with omega-3/omega-6 fatty acids can also produce a false negative test. As a rule, pets should not have been treated with the listed medications for at least 3 to 4 weeks for oral and topical medicines, and 10 to 12 weeks if injectable medicines were administered. At least 10 days should have transpired since the last dose of fatty acids if these have been given to the pet.

Despite the skill required and the potential for inaccurate results, when properly performed, intradermal skin testing is our best method for testing pets suspected to have atopic dermatitis.

## In Vitro Testing

Veterinarians often recommend in vitro (test tube) testing, called blood ELISA or RAST testing, for the diagnosis of atopic dermatitis. There are a number of potential advantages to blood testing: 1) Patients do not require sedation; 2) Much less time is needed to draw blood than to conduct intradermal testing; 3) Medications the pet is taking interfere less with the results (although false negative test results can occur if the pet has been on long-term medical therapy); 4) no special skill is needed to perform the test; and 5) the test can be performed on pets with active skin disease. (Skin testing cannot be performed on pets with active skin disease.)

Despite these potential advantages, there are also disadvantages to in vitro testing. It is not as accurate as intradermal skin testing. Many dogs are incorrectly diagnosed as allergic based upon a false positive blood test. Most dermatologists prefer intradermal skin testing and only use blood testing as a backup. Some dogs who do not respond to antigen therapy based on results from ELISA blood testing may respond to allergens selected based upon intradermal testing. If skin testing is unavailable, the blood test can be used as a screening test as long as the false positive issue is kept in mind. By the way, despite many claims to the contrary, blood testing cannot diagnose food allergies in pets (see page 78–80).

## Skin Biopsy

A skin biopsy can be used in diagnosing atopic dermatitis. A minor surgical procedure performed under heavy sedation or light anesthesia, skin biopsy is an underused method in veterinary medicine. I recommend a skin biopsy when the skin lesions look so strange that I can't even begin to make an educated guess as to what is going on, and in every chronic skin case that comes to me after treatment has gone on for months or years without positive results.

In this procedure, the veterinarian uses a skin punch or scalpel blade to remove several tiny pieces of skin. In most instances, the pieces of removed skin are so small that the incisions do not even require stitches, but can be closed with surgical glue or left open to heal with a small scab. A pathologist examines the tiny pieces of biopsied skin through a microscope, looking for ringworm, mange, immune skin diseases, hormonal diseases, or cancer.

Most of the time, the skin biopsy gives us an exact answer to the pet's problem, so the best treatment can then be selected. In some instances, probably 10 percent of the time, an exact answer is not apparent; the biopsy comes back only with the diagnosis of "chronic proliferative skin disease." In this case, the pathologist saw no infectious or cancerous organisms, or could not identify a specific problem such as hypothyroidism. Sometimes, the pathologist can tell that a hormonal disorder has caused the skin problem. The veterinarian can then test for thyroid disease as well as other hormonal disorders.

There are times when the skin biopsy can be quite helpful in diagnosing atopic dermatitis, as the case of Buddy illustrates.

Buddy is a 12-week-old, mixed-breed male dog his owners acquired from the local animal shelter when he was 8 weeks old. He recently started itching. My physical examination of him showed no obvious cause for the itching; no external parasites such as fleas, lice, or ticks; and no skin lesions such as might occur with ringworm or mange, two very common puppy skin disorders. I prescribed a short dose of corticosteroids and a topical hypoallergenic shampoo and conditioner.

At his recheck 2 weeks later, Buddy's owner reported that the itching had become more severe. There were still no skin lesions or apparent cause for the increased itching. I prescribed a slightly higher dose of corticosteroids and an antihistamine, with instructions to continue the regimen of hypoallergenic shampooing and conditioning.

Two weeks later, Buddy's owner reported that he was still itching, more so now after the treatment of increased corticosteroids and antihistamines that normally relieves the itching if the problem is allergies. At this visit, Buddy exhibited tiny red bumps (papules) on his abdomen and inner thighs. These lesions are often seen in pets with diseases such as bacterial skin infections, fleabite hypersensitivity, and sarcoptic mange. I was tempted to diagnose sarcoptic mange, despite several negative skin scrapings, because Buddy did not respond to increasing doses of corticosteroids and antihistamines and the skin lesions were similar to those seen in pets early in the course of infection with sarcoptic mange. Since both Buddy's owner and I were beginning to lose our patience and wanted to move quickly to help relieve Buddy's obvious distress, I recommended and performed a skin biopsy.

The results of the skin biopsy showed a superficial bacterial infection (the cause of the red bumps) and an underlying allergic dermatitis. Allergies are very rare in puppies Buddy's age, and he certainly did not respond at all to the conventional therapy (corticosteroids and antihistamines) for pets with allergic dermatitis. Before proceeding with any complementary therapies, I knew we needed to get to the bottom of this very challenging case. I referred Buddy to a veterinary dermatologist for a more thorough evaluation which indicated food hypersensitivity. After this consultation, we were able to treat Buddy effectively for his itchy skin by switching him to a hypoallergenic diet. In Buddy's case the skin biopsy allowed us to pinpoint an underlying allergy as the cause of his intense itching.

## Skin Scraping

Skin scraping, one of two basic tests for evaluating skin disease in pets, is used to test for the presence of microscopic mange mites (see chapter 2, page 21). Most dermatologists recommend that this test be performed on most, if not all, cases of skin disease. Even if the skin scraping was performed early in the course of a skin disorder, it should be repeated if the condition becomes chronic, as some cases of mange fail to reveal the mites in the early stages of the disease.

Veterinarians perform skin scraping by placing a drop of mineral oil on the skin, squeezing a small area of skin to express the mites, and scraping the skin with a sterile scalpel blade. As I mentioned in the previous chapter, I prefer to use a glass microscope slide (not the one I put the specimen on) to scrape the skin, due to my concern that I might accidentally cut the animal with the scalpel blade. The doctor then places the scraped material on a glass slide and examines it through a microscope, looking for mites.

It is often difficult to see sarcoptic mange mites (they are only present in the scrapings about 50 percent of the time), so it is necessary to perform skin scrapings from several areas to maximize the chance of finding the mites. Since sarcoptic mange is often difficult to diagnose definitively, I recommend treating for the disease if it is suspected and evaluating the response to treatment to make the diagnosis "in retrospect."

## Fungal Culture

The fungal culture is the second most commonly recommended diagnostic test for pets with skin problems. Fungal culture is performed to look for ringworm (see chapter 2, pages 37–38).

To perform a fungal culture, veterinarians lightly clean the affected area with an alcohol swab to remove surface contamination. They then remove several hairs and crusts from the affected area with forceps and place them on special culture plates. The special plates contain chemicals that inhibit bacterial growth and encourage fungal growth. The plate is placed in a cool dark area and examined daily. Ringworm fungus, if present, grows within 3 to 7 days, producing a white fluffy fungal colony and changing the color of the medium in the culture plates to red. The fluffy colony is then examined microscopically to determine the exact species of ringworm present.

## Wood's Light Examination

The Wood's light examination is another screening test for detecting ringworm infection in pets. The test utilizes an ultraviolet light to examine hairs and scales from affected skin. If ringworm fungus is present, it glows in the dark. The test is only a rough screening test and is not perfect because normal hair and scale may glow in the dark. Also, only

50 percent of ringworm infections caused by a specific type of ringworm, *Microsporum canis,* will glow in the dark. Since there are so many false positive and false negative results, many doctors do not rely on this method as a definitive test for pets with skin disease.

## Skin Cytology

Skin cytology is an underused, but extremely valuable test. I find it to be of most use when looking for secondary yeast infections in dogs with chronic itchy, smelly skin. The test often allows me to diagnose a previously undiagnosed yeast infection and cure what was once a "hopeless" case.

Cytology means examination of cells. Skin cytology involves microscopic examination of the skin. To use this test, the doctor usually rubs a cotton swab on the affected area of skin and then rolls the swab onto a clean microscope slide. The slide is then processed with special stains and examined microscopically for bacteria and yeasts.

## Skin Culture

Culturing the skin is a valuable test in determining proper antibiotic therapy for pets with chronic bacterial dermatitis. Simply culturing the surface of the skin is not adequate; normal skin is loaded with bacteria. If only the skin surface is cultured, many normal bacteria will be identified, which is of no help to the pet.

The only way to get reliable results with a skin culture is to culture pieces of skin obtained through a skin biopsy. The results of the culture will give the identity of bacteria living deep in the dermis of the skin and hair follicles. This skin can also be used to grow the bacteria and create autogenous bacterial vaccines for the specific pet, if this form of therapy is chosen to help the pet with chronic bacterial dermatitis.

## Diet

To diagnose and treat true food allergies, you need to put your dog on a hypoallergenic elimination diet (see chapter 2, pages 43–46). Working with your veterinarian, you may be able to determine if a specific element in your dog's food is causing an allergic response. Once you have identified it, you can eliminate that allergen element from his diet.

If your pet is eating a processed food containing by-products and chemical additives, switching to a more natural diet or, even better, a homemade diet made with fresh ingredients is easy and should be tried at some point during the diagnostic evaluation of your pet.

> To diagnose and treat true food allergies, you need to put your dog on a hypoallergenic elimination diet.

Of course, your dog may have allergic atopic dermatitis in addition to the food allergies you identify. If that is the case, he may improve slightly on an elimination diet, but will still be itchy, necessitating further evaluation. Since diagnosing allergies can be difficult and take months to years, I recommend working with your veterinarian to determine which allergies may be causing your pet to itch.

## Trial Dose of Medical Therapy

Occasionally, veterinarians prescribe medication for the itchy pet to observe the response to the medication. For example, determining if allergies are the cause of a dog's itchiness sometimes involves a great deal of detective work. A doctor might prescribe a trial dose of corticosteroids and observe the pet's response. A positive or negative response to therapy helps identify the cause of the pet's itchiness.

While I don't normally like to use medications as a diagnostic aid, it is sometimes necessary and can provide a wealth of information.

## Diagnostic Imaging: Conventional Radiography (X Rays)

We don't often think of radiography (x rays) as a useful test for pets with skin disease, and most often, it is useless. The one exception is the pet that constantly licks, bites, chews, or rubs one particular area. For example, the dog who always licks one foot might have pain in the foot that could be caused by a fracture or bone tumor. A radiograph would reveal the cause to be an orthopedic problem rather than an allergic disorder.

Early in my practice, I saw an older Miniature Schnauzer that constantly chewed at his hip. Prior therapy for allergies, consisting of corticosteroids, was not helping the poor dog. I sedated him and took a radiograph to look for hip dysplasia or cauda equina syndrome, a spinal disorder. The results were negative for both conditions. My final diagnosis was psychogenic (behavioral) dermatitis, and the dog responded to medical therapy for an obsessive-compulsive disorder. This was long before I started using complementary therapies such as acupuncture and

> Determining if allergies are the cause of a dog's itchiness sometimes involves a great deal of detective work.

herbal therapies, which I could now use to treat a similar problem. The point is that the radiograph is a rarely used but potentially useful tool for those strange cases that just don't seem to be a true dermatological disorder.

Modern x-ray machines are very safe and are calibrated to deliver only the tiny amount of x-ray energy needed to produce high-quality pictures. Most often, the person taking the x-rays takes two views—front-to-back and side-to-side—to allow the doctor to assess perpendicular planes of the involved area.

Since even the best-trained pet will not usually lie still while his body is placed in odd positions, most pets need to be sedated to allow proper positioning and minimize the need for multiple pictures. In some states, anesthesia is required as it is against the law for medical personnel to be in the room when x-rays are taken. Modern sedatives are safe when used properly and the pet is monitored carefully. In my practice, the sedative is reversed with another medication at the completion of the x-ray procedure, and the pet leaves fully awake within minutes after reversal.

## Blood Tests (Basic Blood Count/Profile)

Any pet with chronic skin disease should have a complete blood panel done on him, including several thyroid tests.

A blood count/profile is often used to help the doctor diagnose diseases that might be the cause of the pet's dermatitis, such as thyroid disease. Hypothyroidism, or low thyroid disease, is a common factor in pets with chronic skin disorders. If the blood profile indicates the possibility of thyroid disease, further testing can be conducted. In many cases, thyroid tests are normal yet the pet responds to a trial dose of thyroid medication. Since thyroid medication is safe for dogs when it is prescribed correctly, I often use a trial dose for 4 to 8 weeks to see if the pet shows any response.

Those that do, despite normal blood levels of thyroid hormone, obviously have a problem incorporating thyroid into their cells. In other words, there is a defect at the cellular level, despite normal blood levels of hormone.

When veterinarians suspect an immune cause, such as lupus, in a dog's dermatitis, they may order special immune blood tests. Immune disease rarely causes dermatitis that mimic allergies in pets but, if there is any doubt, your pet's veterinarian might suggest these tests.

Sometimes the blood profile indicates the possibility of a hormonal disease called Cushing's disease. Cushing's disease is a condition in which the adrenal gland overproduces its normal steroid hormones. Dogs with Cushing's disease often overeat, drink too much water, urinate excessively, and experience large amounts of weight gain. These signs resemble those of pets who receive steroid medications for an extended period of time, as well as those pets who have naturally occurring diabetes. Due to the high level of steroid hormone, they are especially prone to infections, most commonly of the bladder or skin.

If Cushing's disease is suspected, based upon physical examination, history, and preliminary blood or urinalysis results, get further testing. These tests can include a urine cortisol test, an ACTH stimulation test, or a low or high dose dexamethasone suppression test. Cushing's disease is often difficult to diagnose, and many cases fall into a "gray" area where firm diagnosis cannot be made. Currently, most doctors recommend that only dogs showing clinical signs of Cushing's disease should be treated regardless of test results. Since dogs with undiagnosed Cushing's disease can suffer chronic recurrent skin infections or be misdiagnosed as allergic, a proper diagnosis is essential to allow the doctor to properly treat these chronic skin infections.

One popular therapy, called orthomolecular therapy uses high doses of antioxidant vitamins and minerals to treat pets with allergies. Since these antioxidants can alter thyroid and adrenal gland testing, it is important to run blood tests for these disorders before beginning antioxidant therapy.

Blood tests also provide information on the general health of the pet, and allow the doctor to determine if alterations in prescribed medications need to be made. For example, a blood test might reveal diabetes. While diabetes does not typically cause skin problems and itching, early detection of this hormonal problem will extend your pet's life by allowing treatment to begin before clinical disease is present.

Since steroidal medications, typically prescribed for pets with atopic dermatitis, can cause intestinal ulcers, kidney disease, increased susceptibility to infections, osteoporosis, and liver disease, it is important to determine if your pet has any of these problems before prescribing the medication. If he does, the doctor may decide to give a lower dose than usual or even use a different medication such as an antihistamine. And since steroidal drugs can also cause these problems, pets that must use these products on a long-term basis (which we hope is very few pets), need to have blood and urine tests every 2 to 3 months to allow early detection of potentially fatal complications from medical therapy.

Once you have determined the cause of your dog's scratching, whether it is atopic dermatitis or another condition, you and your holistic veterinarian can design a proper treatment approach. Often this requires a combination of both conventional and complementary therapies, especially in the difficult chronic cases on which I am often called to consult. In the next chapter, I discuss conventional treatments for atopic dermatitis. In chapter 5, I cover complementary therapy options.

# CHAPTER SUMMARY

- To receive holistic care for your pet, you must locate and consult a holistic veterinarian.

- You and the holistic veterinarian will work together to create the best treatment for your pet.

- Before your appointment, observe your dog carefully so that you can describe all signs and symptoms, but resist giving your dog a bath so that your dog's skin condition can be examined properly.

- Bring your dog's complete medical history and records of previous diagnosis to your appointment.

- In the office, the doctor will perform a complete physical examination of your dog.

- The doctor may run a series of laboratory tests to provide a proper diagnosis.

# ·4·

# Conventional Therapies
# for Atopic Dermatitis

I s there a best treatment for atopic (allergic) dermatitis? In the discussion of conventional treatments in this chapter and the natural therapies in chapter 5, I would like you to consider the following. I believe the "perfect" treatment for allergies should meet these criteria:

1. The treatment should be cost effective.
2. The treatment should be easy for the owner to administer.
3. The treatment must be safe for the pet.
4. The treatment must have minimal or no short- and long-term side effects.
5. The treatment should ideally help control the cause of the problem, rather than just cover up the clinical signs of scratching.

No matter what approach you ultimately choose, it should meet as many of these conditions as possible to be of most benefit to your pet. As you will soon see, complementary treatments fill most of these requirements, whereas conventional medications do not and are rarely suitable as the long-term treatment for most allergic dogs.

Along with the criteria for a perfect treatment, keep in mind that no type of treatment, conventional or complementary, should be administered on a long-term basis without a proper diagnosis. The following case is a classic example of failing to diagnose the disease and then administering an incorrect treatment.

The owners of Pasha, a 5-year-old female Golden Retriever, brought her to me for evaluation. The previous doctor had prescribed monthly steroid methylprednisolone injections for Pasha's scratching, which he suspected was the result of atopic dermatitis. The owner told me that this doctor had not done any diagnostic testing to arrive at this diagnosis of allergic dermatitis, despite the fact that Pasha showed signs of hair loss and had several tiny red bumps (papules) on her skin. Most allergic dogs simply itch a lot, but their skin appears normal, except when they have secondary infections.

My examination of Pasha showed extensive areas of hair loss and numerous papules. Her skin lesions led me to believe that she was suffering from something more serious than allergies. Since there were no signs of fleas on Pasha, a common cause of this type of lesion in dogs in my practice area, I suspected a disease process occurring deeper in her skin.

I performed a skin scraping, a simple test used to detect the presence of mange mites (see chapter 3, page 73). Any doctor can easily perform this test. It should be used in the diagnosis of most, if not all, skin cases; especially those like Pasha's, where the pet is not getting better despite what appears to be the correct treatment.

The skin scrapings showed demodectic mange. This type of mange usually occurs in puppies. When it occurs in older pets, it is often the result of an underlying problem that indicates a compromised immune system. Therefore, I checked blood and urine specimens from Pasha, which were normal.

I suspected that the incorrect treatment of her itching had caused Pasha to break out with this case of mange. Steroids should rarely if ever be used in pets suspected of having demodectic mange because steroids suppress the immune system, which can allow mange mites to overgrow and cause terrible problems. (Steroids can be safely used in cases of sarcoptic mange, as the mites that cause this type of mange have nothing to do with a defective immune system.)

I took Pasha off the steroids and treated her mange with conventional dips, homeopathy, and nutritional therapies. Within 6 weeks, Pasha was back to normal.

In this case, Pasha's original skin lesions and increased itchiness after treatment should have prompted the original doctor to obtain a correct

> An important part of the holistic treatment for allergic pets includes obtaining the proper diagnosis as soon as possible so that the correct treatment can be safely administered to your dog.

diagnosis. I often diagnose demodectic mange in pets incorrectly treated with corticosteroids. These pets suffer needlessly and their owners spend money unnecessarily, all because the original doctor failed to perform a simple diagnostic test and institute the correct treatment. An important part of the holistic treatment for allergic pets includes obtaining the proper diagnosis as soon as possible so that the correct treatment can be safely administered to your dog.

# Conventional Treatments

The most commonly prescribed conventional treatment for allergies is corticosteroids (steroids). The second most common is antihistamines. While these medications can be effective in controlling itching in allergic patients, they do nothing to correct or cure the underlying disorder. All too often they are prescribed for chronic, long-term control of allergies without searching for safer alternatives. As a result, many pets suffer unnecessary side effects from these treatments and never seem to stop scratching.

> Any approach you select should help minimize the inflammation and discomfort that causes your dog to scratch. Thinking holistically, you must also consider the overall health of the dog.

In the following chapter, you'll learn about a number of therapies that holistic veterinarians like myself use to help control the itching and inflammation that plague allergic pets. At this point, I want to review the conventional treatments, point out the potential side effects (which will reveal why it is imperative to search for safer long-term therapies for your pet), and teach you how these conventional treatments can be used safely and effectively when needed to provide short-term relief from the itchiness that bothers so many allergic dogs.

# A CLOSER LOOK

Cell membranes contain chemicals called phospholipids. When the cell membrane is injured, as in the allergic pet, an enzyme acts on the phospholipids to produce the fatty acids arachidonic acid (an omega-6 fatty acid) and eicosapentaenoic acid (an omega-3 fatty acid). Further metabolism of these two fatty acids by additional enzymes yields the production of chemicals called eicosanoids.

The eicosanoids produced by metabolism of arachidonic acid (omega-6) are pro-inflammatory (meaning they cause inflammation), suppress the immune system, and cause platelets to aggregate and clot. The eicosanoids produced by metabolism of eicosapentaenoic acid (omega-3) are non-inflammatory, not immunosuppressive, and help inhibit platelets from clotting.

The various drugs used in allergy treatment work at different stages to help decrease the production of the pro-inflammatory compounds. For example, corticosteroids work at two places in this biochemical pathway. They help inhibit the enzyme that is responsible for metabolizing the membrane phospholipids into arachidonic and eicosapentaenoic acids, and they inhibit the enzyme responsible for breaking down arachidonic acid into pro-inflammatory compounds.

Remember that atopic dermatitis is an inflammatory, uncomfortable condition. As a result, any approach you select should help minimize the inflammation and discomfort that causes your dog to scratch. Thinking holistically, you must also consider the overall health of the dog.

Some of our conventional treatments are potentially harmful to the pet when used as the sole long-term therapy for treating allergies. For example, many doctors choose long-term therapy with corticosteroids for pets with atopic dermatitis. While corticosteroids will relieve inflammation and itching, they do nothing to try and help the immune system to counteract the allergies. And with the long-term side effects associated with corticosteroids, this choice of treatment is too risky unless absolutely necessary. Although the dog will feel better for a while, the treatment is actually making his health worse.

### Understanding Inflammation

Inflammation is caused by damage to the tissues and cells of the affected body part. When a tissue is inflamed, it exhibits any or all of the following signs: redness, pain, tenderness, swelling, and loss of function. See "A Closer Look" (page 87) for the biochemical mechanisms of inflammation.

Let's take a look at the two most common classes of medications currently used to treat atopic dermatitis.

# CORTICOSTEROIDS

CORTICOSTEROIDS, OR STEROIDS for short, are the first class of medication that comes to mind when thinking of treating the allergic dog. The reason steroids are used in the treatment of allergic dogs is that they work extremely well and very quickly. For most pets, the scratching, redness of the skin, and inflammation are relieved within 24 hours of taking steroids.

While steroids can be used safely and intelligently in a holistic approach to help allergic pets, they are one of the most frequently used and abused drugs in veterinary and probably human medicine. It's just too easy for doctors to reach for the magic "steroid shot" to treat symptoms, without diagnosing and treating the disease. As a result, pets are often incorrectly treated for months or years before someone says, "Enough. There must be a better way!"

Many holistic-minded people think that corticosteroids are horrible drugs that are to be avoided at all costs. That is far from the truth, however. When a diagnosis suggests a disease that is most correctly treated with corticosteroids, they are actually wonderful drugs that often can be lifesaving. Steroids must be used correctly, at the right dose, for the proper length of time, and in the right patient. The problem is that this is often not the case.

> While steroids can be used safely and intelligently in a holistic approach to help allergic pets, they are one of the most frequently used and abused drugs in veterinary and probably human medicine.

Due to their numerous short-term and long-term side effects, they have no place in the management of the pet with chronic allergies, except in the rarest of pets where no other treatment gives the animal relief and the alternative is euthanasia. However, rational short term use of corticosteroids (to quickly relieve inflammation and

# A CLOSER LOOK

Just what are corticosteroids? Why do so many in the health-care field seem so eager to use these miracle drugs? Corticosteroids, or more correctly glucocorticoids, are hormones produced by the adrenal glands under the control of the pituitary gland. When the body needs to produce more of its own glucocorticoids, the pituitary gland produces a hormone called adrenocorticotrophic hormone (ACTH) that stimulates the adrenal gland to produce more glucocorticoids. When the level of glucocorticoids rises, the pituitary shuts off its signal (ACTH) to the adrenal gland. When the level of glucocorticoids falls, the pituitary puts out more ACTH. This loop keeps the body's production of glucocorticoids in check with the body's demand.

When the dog receives corticosteroids as a treatment, his pituitary gland senses this and stops production of ACTH so the adrenal glands won't make any more steroid. This effectively shuts down the body's normal production of a vitally important hormone. This won't hurt the pet if a low dose of steroid is administered for a short period of time, say 7 to 10 days. More potent steroids provided for longer periods of time, such as those once-a-month shots so often given to allergic pets, represent a potent depot (long-lasting) form of the drug. Suddenly stopping the steroids after chronic use can cause serious withdrawal problems because the dog's body can't adapt that quickly to pick up the production of steroids again. This is one of the potentially serious side effects that occurs when pets are treated with steroids.

itching) can be part of a holistic treatment regimen for the allergic dog.

## What Corticosteroids Do

As I mentioned, corticosteroids do a number of wonderful things. First, they are anti-inflammatory, analgesic (pain-relieving), and antipruritic (itch-relieving). They decrease inflammation, swelling, pain caused by inflammation, and itching. They are also very helpful in the initial treatment of patients with severe shock and neurological disease, as they relieve inflammation in spinal cord and brain injuries.

The negative side of these wonderful effects is that they can decrease the ability of wounds to heal and increase the chance of infection (if used for too long or at high doses; pets that must have long-term steroid therapy need careful, frequent monitoring to allow for early detection of infections). For pets with arthritis, they contribute to further destruction of arthritic joints by decreasing collagen and proteoglycan synthesis, making them a poor choice for long-term therapy for most pets with arthritis.

At a high enough dose, corticosteroids are also immuno-suppressive, which means they suppress the body's immune system. While this can be useful in immune diseases where the body is attacking itself, as stated before, an animal with a suppressed immune system is more prone to infections (including skin infections, which are often seen in allergic patients).

## Side Effects of Corticosteroids

There are many more short- and long-term side effects of steroids you should know about before consenting to use these medications on your allergic pet. Corticosteroids cause an increase in appetite, an increase in water intake, and an increase in urine output. These side effects are commonly observed in most, if not all, dogs on corticosteroid therapy. Even those pets taking the medications for a short time and at a very low dose can exhibit these side effects. The higher the dose and the longer the therapy, the worse the problems. While these side effects are not harmful per se, they are upsetting to many owners. Therefore, when using corticosteroids as part of the treatment of the allergic dog, it is preferable to give the lowest doses possible for the shortest amount of time.

The side effects of long-term use are a totally different story. Long-term corticosteroid treatment affects nearly every organ of a dog's body, leading to serious damage to your pet's quality of life. In addition, the use of steroids upsets laboratory tests, making artificial changes in liver enzymes, white blood cell values, and thyroid tests that may cause the misdiagnosis of other problems. Steroids can also have serious interactions with other prescription drugs, including Phenobarbital, Lasix (furosemide), digoxin, and NSAIDS (Rimadyl, EctoGesic).

Both the short- and long-term use of corticosteroids alter adrenal and thyroid hormone levels in the blood. I recommend that blood be tested 4 to 8 weeks after stopping steroid therapy to diagnose any side effects that might have occurred as a result of chronic steroid therapy. A long-acting steroid shot can last 6 to 8 weeks after the injection; in this case, blood should be tested after the effects of the steroid shot have worn off, usually 8 weeks after the injection.

Since the side effects of long-term corticosteroid therapy are numerous and serious, I prefer not to use steroids any more than absolutely necessary. Pets on long-term therapy must be monitored for side effects. Monitoring includes physical examination and blood and urine tests every 2 to 3 months.

# SIDE EFFECTS OF LONG-TERM CORTICOSTEROID USE IN DOGS

The following are some of the side effects long-term corticosteroid therapy can have on your dog:

1. Heart and cardiovascular system problems causing hypertension (high blood pressure) and sodium and water retention

2. Kidney and liver diseases

3. Skin irritation causing acne, infections, excessive bruising, degeneration or thinning of the skin, and hair loss

4. Hormonal and reproductive irregularity resulting in infertility, growth failure, adrenal gland diseases, birth defects, and spontaneous abortion

5. Gastrointestinal problems including GI bleeding, ulcers, pancreatitis, and perforation

6. Immune system suppression, decreased ability to resist infections, anemia, and low blood platelet counts

7. Metabolic imbalance resulting in increased blood fat, fatty liver disease, and obesity

8. Musculoskeletal weakness leading to osteoporosis, muscle weakness, and possible cartilage destruction

9. Behavioral problems leading to aggression, depression, hyperactivity, and lethargy

10. Eye problems leading to glaucoma and cataracts

11. Respiratory issues including thromboembolism or blood clots in the lungs

12. Neurologic disease such as seizures, paralysis, and unsteadiness

# DURATION OF COMMONLY USED CORTICOSTEROIDS

The actual duration of a corticosteroid, meaning how long a dose exerts its effects in the body, depends upon a number of factors, including the specific formulation of the medication. For example, the acetate and acetonide formulations of corticosteroids are repositol, or very long-acting, preparations that can act for weeks and last in the body for several months. These preparations are overused in veterinary medicine and are the most harmful if used repeatedly.

**Short acting:** Duration 8–12 hours
- Hydrocortisone

**Intermediate acting:** Duration 12–36 hours
- Prednisone
- Prednisolone
- Methylprednisolone (Solu-Delta)
- Triamcinolone

**Long acting:** Duration longer than 36 hours
- Betamethasone
- Dexamethasone (Azium)

Due to the side effects, pets on long-term corticosteroid therapy, as a rule, are not expected to live as long as if they were not on these medications. This is why it is so distressing to see pets with allergies sentenced to a shortened life of corticosteroid therapy when no other therapies have ever been tried. Sure, there are those very rare pets that do not respond to any conventional treatment or complementary therapy so must take corticosteroids for life. And with appropriate dosing and monitoring, even these pets can have a decent quality of life if doctors are careful in their handling of these cases. Sadly, it's too easy for doctors and owners to give up and reach for the steroids any time a pet itches. I choose long-term therapy with corticosteroids for the allergic pet only if all other safer approaches have failed after a year of trying and only if my other choice is euthanasia.

> Sadly, it's too easy for doctors and owners to give up and reach for the steroids any time a pet itches.

My intention in relating all of these facts to you is not to scare you into avoiding corticosteroids altogether, but rather to educate you. When it comes to treating allergic skin disease, there are definitely better choices than settling for long-term, high-dose corticosteroid therapy. For those pets that may require corticosteroids or for those owners who want to use them on a short-term basis, I prefer to use a lower dose of corticosteroids when owners agree to try nutritional supplements and other more natural therapies for pets with allergies. These therapies, discussed in the next

## A CLOSER LOOK

The side effect of sedation from antihistamines in both people and pets is related to individual susceptibility. Some patients are more likely to experience this side effect than others are. Sedation also has to do with the type of antihistamine. So-called first-generation antihistamines (such as hydroxyzine, diphenhydramine, and chlorpheniramine) enter the central nervous system and brain quite easily, and cause sedation. Second-generation antihistamines (such as loratidine and terfenadine) do not enter the central nervous system as easily and are less likely to cause sedation. On the other hand, terfenadine has been reported to cause serious heart arrhythmias in people. This is most likely to occur in those with liver disease or low blood magnesium or potassium, and when terfenadine is used with drugs such as ketoconazole, itraconazole, and erythromycin. This is probably true for dogs as well as humans, although use of terfenadine is uncommon in pets, and the three drugs mentioned that negatively interact with it are unlikely to be used (although it's possible).

chapter, often allow us to use lower doses of the more potent corticosteroids.

## ANTIHISTAMINES

ANTIHISTAMINES REPRESENT THE second class of medications often recommended to decrease itching in the allergic pet. For long-term use, antihistamines are preferable to corticosteroids because they have fewer side effects.

Histamine is a chemical released by mast cells and basophil cells in the pet's body in response to contact with the allergen (foreign substance such as mold, ragweed, grass protein, etc.). Histamine "locks onto" histamine receptors (H1 receptors) located on various cells throughout the body. Think of histamine as a key that fits into its receptor, which acts as the lock. When histamine locks onto the receptor, the cell undergoes biochemical changes and produces the clinical signs associated with allergies, such as itching and runny eyes and nose. The histamine receptors also cause increased permeability of blood vessels (resulting in edema or fluid formation), the release of other chemicals that increase inflammation, and an accumulation of inflammatory cells.

> Only trial and error can determine whether an antihistamine will help reduce the pet's need for corticosteroids.

Antihistamines work by blocking the histamine receptors. In so doing, the antihistamines physically prevent histamine from connecting with its receptor, preventing the clinical signs mentioned above. A number of studies have tested the effectiveness of various antihistamines in treating allergies in pets. The results have been variable, with anywhere from 10 percent to 30 percent of dogs showing improvement.

Antihistamines are not as effective in controlling signs seen in allergic pets as are corticosteroids. This is because antihistamines function by blocking the histamine receptors

# COMMON ANTIHISTAMINES

Benadryl (diphenhydramine)
Chlortrimeton (chlorpheniramine)
Atarax/Vistaryl (hydroxyzine)
Tavist (clemastine)
Seldane (terfenadine)*
Periactin (cyproheptadine)
Temaril (trimeprazine)
Hismanal (astemizole)*
Claritine (loratadine)*

* Terfenadine, astemizole, and loratadine were ineffective in several animal studies, but your veterinarian may try them at various dosages if the more common antihistamines do not offer the pet relief.

on cells in the body; whereas corticosteroids function by preventing the formation of prostaglandins and other chemicals that cause itching as well as by stabilizing allergy cells to prevent them from "breaking apart" and releasing their chemical mediators of inflammation. Also keep in mind that histamine is only one of many chemicals released by allergy cells (mast cells). This means that all of the other chemicals released upon contact with the allergen remain free to cause itching even though histamine may be prevented from doing so. Additionally, antihistamines work best to prevent itching before allergy signs are evident; they are not as effective in decreasing itching once the pet is severely itchy.

The response to antihistamines varies in pets. In some dogs, none of the choices of antihistamines produce any effect. In other patients, the first antihistamine tried works great! There is no way to predict which antihistamine will work on which pet. Only trial and error can determine that, as well as whether an antihistamine will help reduce the pet's need for corticosteroids.

The major side effect in dogs taking antihistamines is sedation (sleepiness). Naturally, this is much less of a problem in pets than in people. If sedation occurs, it will of course decrease the dog's itching just because he is too sedated to itch! Long-term sedation is not desirable, however. In some cases, the sedation wears off in a few days. If this does not occur, your veterinarian can lower the dosage, increase the dosing interval, or try another antihistamine.

There is no data on the long-term safety of antihistamines, but experience seems to indicate they are relatively safe and much more so than corticosteroids if chronic drug therapy is required.

Since antihistamines are metabolized by the liver, they should be used cautiously in pets with liver disease. They should not be used, unless absolutely necessary, in pets with glaucoma, urinary retention disorders, or intestinal atony, a disorder involving a lack of intestinal tone. Antihistamines can cause birth defects, so should not be used in pregnant animals.

# HYPOSENSITIZATION

FOR THOSE PETS that do not respond to other conventional therapies, hyposensitization may be necessary. Hyposensitization involves weekly injections of antigens (foreign proteins to which the dog has exhibited allergies), which are commonly referred to as allergy shots. After skin testing to determine the exact protein that affects the dog, the doctor compounds a solution containing that allergen. The idea is that the dog's body will be sensitized to the protein and experience fewer allergic signs upon the next exposure to the allergen.

It may surprise you when I mention that antigen injections are actually a somewhat "homeopathic" approach to treating the pet with atopic dermatitis. Many people think of allergy shots as only a conventional medicine, but think about it. Homeopathy stimulates the body to heal itself. While it doesn't use shots to deliver its medicine, the remedies (in pill form) are diluted solutions of products that in stronger amounts would actually cause the disease. With conventional allergy shots, diluted amounts of foreign proteins (allergens) are used to get the body not to respond in an allergic way, but rather in a healing way.

That said, I try to avoid hyposensitization if at all possible. First, it is rarely necessary as most pets respond to the various complementary therapies listed in this book. Second, there are potential side effects of hyposensitization, including allergic reactions to the injected antigens. Third, antigen injections are expensive, although by no means cost-prohibitive for most owners. Fourth, it takes at least 12 months to determine if the pet is responding to the injections. This means the dog requires other forms of care for an entire year while you and your veterinarian wait to see if hyposensitization will work. Fifth, only about 70 percent of pets respond favorably to hyposensitization, meaning that 30 percent of the dogs treated are still horribly allergic at the end of the trial year.

I only use hyposensitization under two circumstances. In the first circumstance, I've tried everything possible, but the dog has not improved and requires very high doses of corticosteroids to even survive with its allergic disorder. The second circumstance is when the owner wants to pursue that therapy. Some owners do not have the patience or interest in trying a number of complementary therapies for their allergic pets. In a few cases, the owners I see are fed up with frequent veterinary visits, trying one drug after another, and dealing with pets that itch and smell. Some are literally at their wit's end! For those clients who no longer have the interest or patience to wait and see if complementary therapies will help their pets, I do not hesitate to refer their dog to a dermatologist for skin testing and antigen therapy. I encourage them to keep trying some of my suggested holistic approaches as hyposensitization will require 12 more months of their patience before they know if this therapy is effective for their dog!

## How Hyposensitization Works

We're not really sure why hyposensitization works, but there are several theories. Perhaps it causes reduced levels of IgE. Remember that IgE antibodies bind to the allergens and mast cells and cause the pet to itch. It may be that desensitization of allergic cells reduces the reactivity of mast and other allergic cells. Then again, immunization may be the mechanism, much like vaccination, in which a different class of antibodies, possibly IgG, is formed instead of IgE. Another theory is the development of tolerance as the body forms allergen-specific suppressor cells that suppress the allergic response. Of course, it could be a combination of any or all of these theories.

If you elect to try hyposensitization on your dog, be sure that he is properly diagnosed and that the antigen therapy is based on accurate skin testing. You also should at the very least improve your pet's diet and begin nutritional supplements and topical decontamination. These latter ideas and other complementary therapy approaches are discussed in the next chapter.

# CHAPTER SUMMARY

- Be sure your pet has received a proper diagnosis before accepting any treatment approach.

- A holistic approach may include both conventional treatments and complementary therapies.

- Atopic dermatitis causes inflammation that leads to itchiness and scratching.

- The most common conventional treatment for atopic dermatitis is the use of corticosteroids.

- The second most common conventional treatment for atopic dermatitis is the use of antihistamines.

- Hyposensitization, also called antigen therapy or allergy shots, involves the injection of a diluted allergen; it should be tried only if other therapies fail.

# ·5·

# Complementary Therapies for Atopic Dermatitis

A s PEOPLE TURN to more natural, holistic care for their own bodies, many are choosing the same approach for their pets. In my practice, three approaches—topical treatments, nutritional and other supplements such as fatty acids and antioxidants, and proper diet—form the foundation for treating atopic dermatitis. In many cases, these three alone are so effective that I don't need to turn to the herbs, acupuncture, or homeopathic remedies that also may be effective in the treatment of allergies in dogs. Success with these complementary approaches allows us to lower or eliminate the need for corticosteroids or antihistamines except for the occasional flare-ups that occur as the seasons change.

You must keep in mind that many allergic pets will never be entirely itch free. Success may mean that your dog is "comfortably itchy." Success may mean that you resort to steroids or antihistamines, but only on an infrequent basis. Or it may mean that you use these medications on your dog more often, but in decreased amounts.

Take the cases of Fred and Ethel. Fred is a dog who was receiving monthly injections of the long-acting steroid methylprednisolone to control his itching. After eight months of trying various supplements, I found a successful balance, Fred's scratching decreased, and we were able to discontinue his steroid injections. Now his owner administers short-acting oral prednisone only on an as-needed basis, usually just for a few days whenever his allergies flare up in the spring and fall.

Ethel is another dog that was receiving monthly steroid injections to lessen her scratching. In her case, months of nutritional therapy lead to a lessening of her scratching and the elimination of the harmful injections. Her owner still has to give Ethel oral prednisone every 2 to 3 days to make her comfortably itchy, however. While this was not the complete success we hope for, these short-acting steroids are much safer for Ethel than the injections she had received for years.

In both cases, the dogs and their owners achieved "success," but the ultimate maintenance therapy differed for each pet. While I love to be able to totally wean pets off of all medications, this is not always practical. Success is different for each patient.

There is a wide range of complementary therapies, but it is beyond the scope of this book to examine each one in detail. Therefore, I will concentrate on the most popular ones. Keep in mind that several different types of complementary therapies are often used simultaneously to maximize the chance of a successful outcome. Using multiple complementary approaches can also decrease the need for conventional treatments. There's no way I can prescribe what you should use for your pet, since each pet has individual needs. I suggest that you emphasize the holistic approach and work with your veterinarian to determine which approach is best for your scratching dog.

# Topical Treatments

Avoiding allergens is extremely important when caring for the allergic pet. Several avoidance techniques are discussed in chapter 8. While you can't keep your dog away from every allergen in his environment, you need to remove the allergens he has contact with as quickly as possible. Frequent bathing and conditioning is probably the most important part of the treatment of the allergic dog. Remember that your dog absorbs a lot of allergens through his skin. When you can remove these allergens, you decrease the exposure to the trigger that causes the dog to itch. When he itches less, he scratches less. Even pets on high doses of corticosteroids need frequent bathing and conditioning to remove the things from their bodies that cause itching.

## Bathing Frequency

How often is "frequent"? Each pet will require a different regimen, but in general shampoo and condition your dog every other day or 2 to 3 times per week during the allergic season. Once the scratching is under control, decrease the bathing and conditioning to an as-needed regimen, which is usually once a week. For a severely allergic dog, consider daily bathing until he is comfortable, then weaning to 1 to 2 times per week to maintain a "comfortably itchy" pet.

Are you surprised by this recommendation? Many people have been conditioned to the concept that bathing too often is bad for dogs and dries out their skin. While frequent bathing of a healthy dog with harsh, soapy shampoos can dry out and irritate the skin, the allergic dog has a disease that requires frequent bathing and conditioning. If you use gentle shampoos and conditioners, it is only the rare pet that develops dry, itchy skin. This can easily be remedied by adding a bath oil to the final rinse, but it is rarely needed. In fact, most allergic dogs improve considerably with frequent use of a hypoallergenic shampoo and conditioner.

## Use Hypoallergenic Shampoos and Conditioners

You can use a number of products to bathe and condition the coat and skin of allergic pets. I like to start with the mildest product first, and use more medicated products only as needed. What do we mean by the term "hypoallergenic" shampoo and conditioner? First, any shampoo or conditioner can irritate a pet's skin. Those designated as "hypoallergenic" are least likely to do that. The shampoo and conditioner serve to remove allergens from your dog's skin and hair, condition and rehydrate the skin, reduce flakiness (flaky skin is itchy skin), and decrease inflammation and itching. The "ideal" hypoallergenic shampoo and conditioner should:

- **Be soap free.** Soap can irritate and dry the skin, especially when the pet is bathed frequently, which is necessary when trying to decontaminate the allergic pet. Hypoallergenic shampoos use surfactants to remove the dirt and excess oil on the skin and coat.

- **Be easy to use.** It's hard enough to find time to bathe and condition your pets several times each week. The product must be easy to apply and rinse off.

- **Contain anti-itching ingredients.** The most common holistic ingredient is colloidal oatmeal. I prescribe a product that contains the oatmeal plus aloe vera, which is known for its healing, soothing, and anti-inflammatory properties.

- **Look and smell nice.** I know it seems odd to mention this, but keep in mind that if you don't like the way the product looks or smells, you probably won't use it very often, if at all. All things being equal, I choose products that are attractive looking and smelling.

## Consider Medicated Shampoos and Conditioners

Your veterinarian may recommend other types of shampoos for your dog. For an allergic pet that does not respond to the mild hypoallergenic shampoos, you can use a medicated shampoo and/or leave-on conditioner to decrease his itching. These are basically hypoallergenic products that contain topical anesthetics, antihistamines, or corticosteroids. Obviously, when we're trying to find a natural approach to treating itching, we'd prefer not to use medicated products. However, using a topical product containing medication such as antihistamines or corticosteroids is preferable to using these drugs orally or by injection. If your dog requires such a product and the product decreases the itching without the use of oral medications, seriously consider such an approach. Anything we can do to decrease the need for oral or injected drugs is important.

> Anything we can do to decrease the need for oral or injected drugs is important.

Other types of medicated shampoos and conditioners include those designed for pets with infections. Since so many allergic dogs have skin infections, you might need to use these products for short-term treatment.

While frequent hypoallergenic shampooing and conditioning are an extremely important part—maybe *the most important* part—of the treatment of the itchy dog, the majority of pets do not improve with shampooing and conditioning alone. You should use these topical applications as one part of your pet's treatment. When combined with nutritional supplements, feeding a natural diet, and other complementary therapies, shampooing and conditioning can be quite effective in removing foreign proteins from the skin and coat of the dog, relieving itching, and assisting the skin in healing.

### Glycoproteins

As with so many complementary therapies, there are a number of anecdotal reports showing that treating dogs with atopic dermatitis topically with glycoproteins (a sugar-protein molecule) produced relief from itching and inflammation. Research is needed to provide a better idea of just how glycoproteins work and how they are effective.

Aloe vera is the main source of a glycoprotein called acemannan. Look for either aloe vera or acemannan as an ingredient in shampoos and conditioners. It is in the brand that I prescribe for pets with atopic dermatitis, along with colloidal oatmeal, which is also well known for its topical anti-itching effect.

# NUTRITIONAL SUPPLEMENTS

THERE ARE A number of nutritional supplements that may be beneficial for the allergic dog. Commonly used supplements include enzymes, green foods, fatty acids, and health formulas that contain antioxidants. Any of these supplements can be useful by themselves or in combination with other approaches. Many pet owners giving their dogs nutri-

# A CLOSER LOOK

The true biologic mechanisms explaining how acemannan, ambrotose, and other glycoproteins work to help heal wounds, relieve inflammation, and modulate the immune system have not been clearly defined. Acemannan has been shown to increase the body's production of immune-modulating chemicals, including interleukins 1 and 6 and tumor necrosis factor. These chemicals are quite helpful in shrinking solid sarcoma tumors, for which one acemannan product has been approved for use in pets. These chemicals are pro-inflammatory, however; studies in people have shown them to be involved in the increase in inflammation in people with atopic dermatitis. It does not make sense that they would be useful in treating atopic pets, but there are anecdotal reports in the literature showing effectiveness in some pets. Since acemannan can increase the ability of the white blood cells to destroy microbes, it can be helpful in pets with skin infections. Also, acemannan (and many other natural supplements) probably has other properties that have not yet been defined that can account for its ability to relieve itching and inflammation in atopic pets. Some product literature hints that the ingredients might support cellular communication. Good communication between cells is necessary for proper gland and organ function, proper system function, and optimal health.

tional supplements are able to reduce the dose of steroids or antihistamines. Our ultimate goal is to wean the animals off of all medications.

There is no "ideal" supplement and supplements are not cure-alls. No one supplement is perfect for every pet in every situation. Deciding which supplement to use is not easy. As a veterinarian, I certainly have favorite products that I have used with success in a variety of medical conditions. You should know that there is no one "best" product for helping pets with atopic dermatitis. If one product doesn't produce the desired effect, your doctor has a choice of other products to try. When a supplement is used as directed, there are usually no side effects, unless the product contains drugs or chemical fillers.

> Many pet owners giving their dogs nutritional supplements are able to reduce the dose of steroids or antihistamines.

Do not expect overnight results. Expect to give a product to your dog for at least two months to determine if it is effective. Usually, I recommend starting the supplement at a higher dose (often double the maintenance dose) for 4 to 6 weeks, and then lowering the dose to the maintenance dose when you see results. Some of these products are expensive, especially for larger dogs, but decreasing the dose to the lowest effective amount for maintenance reduces your costs. While we're waiting to see if we get positive results, the pet may need another form of therapy for immediate relief from itching and control inflammation. Acupuncture, homeopathy, and even short-term use of corticosteroids can be helpful for that.

Using several different types of supplements simultaneously can maximize the chance of a successful outcome and decrease the need for conventional drug therapy. Work with your veterinarian to determine which course of therapy is best for your dog.

Occasionally, despite considerable improvement, some dogs experience particularly bad days. This most often occurs as the pollen seasons change and environmental allergens increase. Conventional therapy, acupuncture, or homeopathy can also be useful during these bad days. This trend is typical and does not indicate a failure of your maintenance program of feeding a proper diet, giving nutritional supplements, and bathing and conditioning your dog regularly with hypoallergenic products.

Expect to try several supplements before you obtain a positive response. Commonly, I use multiple supplements to get an additive effect and produce

> Expect to give a product to your dog for at least two months to determine if it is effective.

results. It may take 2 to 3 months before we achieve a good balance and see positive effects. Your dog's body needs time to detoxify from prior treatment before it can begin assimilating the nutrients that produce improvement.

Since the supplement industry is young and not stringently regulated, you should only use nutritional supplements under veterinary supervision. As you consider nutritional supplements, keep in mind that an "ideal" supplement should:

- **Be safe** and not harm your pet.

- **Taste good** to your dog. It must be palatable so that your pet will ingest it.

- **Be cost effective.** Of course, if the supplement can prevent or cure disease, you will save money in veterinary expenses over the life of your pet.

- **Be easy for you to administer.** Many medications that doctors prescribe are never given to the pet because the owner experiences difficulty in administering it. Supplements come in the form of a pill, liquid, chewable tablet, or powder to be sprinkled on the pet's food. The powdered form may be the easiest to give pets.

- **Not interfere with other therapies** that may be necessary for the pet.

- **Have a known dosage.** The requirement of a known correct dosage is the one requirement of the ideal nutritional supplement that is the hardest to meet. Anecdotal evidence and clinical experience rather than hard scientific studies are the bases on which many supplements are recommended. This doesn't mean the supplements are not effective. Many of those for which the "best" dosage is not known are used safely and effectively in dogs with atopic dermatitis. Since studies with specific dosages are often lacking for the use of many supplements, you must work closely with your doctor to review the available supplements and try to find the most appropriate dosage possible. When supplements fail to work, it may be simply that the dosage was off.

As I have said, there is much anecdotal evidence on the effectiveness of many nutritional supplements in the treatment of a variety of disorders in pets, but controlled scientific studies are often lacking. Holistic doctors like myself have no problem trying products based on anecdotal information, but we encourage additional scientific studies to determine the true effectiveness of any complementary therapy. More research is needed on enzymes, green foods, fatty acids, and health blend formulas in the treatment of atopic dermatitis. I encourage you to talk with your pet's doctor about trying supplements. While they are safe and without side effects, you want to be sure that the doctor is aware of every aspects of your dog's treatment.

## Enzymes

Cellular processes, digestion, and absorption of dietary nutrients depend upon the presence of the proper enzymes. The pancreas produces the enzymes amylase, lipase, and various proteases. Amylase breaks down carbohydrates, lipase breaks down fats, and proteases break down proteins. Once pancreatic enzymes properly "digest" these foods, the body can absorb the dietary nutrients they contain. In some atopic dogs, the increased absorption of nutrients helps to relieve itching and inflammation. Enzymes may also enable absorption of as yet undetermined dietary nutrients (perhaps important phytonutrients, natural plant chemicals with possible medicinal effects) that aid in the healing of the skin.

> Even pets on natural raw diets can benefit from additional enzymes, which is why veterinarians often recommend them as a supplement.

## A CLOSER LOOK

Another enzyme of value for allergic conditions is glutathione peroxidase. Glutathione peroxidase is important in breaking down various chemicals (leukotrienes, by-products of arachidonic acid) involved in prompting allergic reactions. Glutathione peroxidase is dependent upon the antioxidant mineral selenium. In asthmatic people, there is evidence of decreased levels of glutathione peroxidase. Giving extra selenium in the form of a natural vitamin-mineral supplement or plant enzyme supplement (which increases selenium absorption) may increase the level of glutathione peroxidase. This helps control leukotrienes and thus allergic reactions.

While it is true that the pancreas produces enzymes to aid in food digestion, additional enzymes found in the diet contribute to digestion and absorption as well. Natural, raw diets contain a number of chemicals, including enzymes, not found in processed foods. Enzymes are destroyed by low (freezing) and high (120 to 160°F) temperatures, so processing food depletes it of enzymes, as well as nutrients. If your pet's diet consists of processed, packaged food, even the more natural kind, he is not getting any enzymes to aid in digestion and his pancreas must supply them all. Giving your dog enzyme supplements can remedy this. Even pets on natural raw diets can benefit from additional enzymes, which is why veterinarians often recommend them as a supplement.

Enzymes work by liberating essential nutrients from the pet's diet. This means that they work best when the pet is eating the best, most healthy and natural diet possible. While we don't know all the wonderful things that enzymes do, we do know that certain enzyme supplements can increase the absorption of essential vitamins, minerals, and fatty acids from the diet. Research has detected increased absorption of zinc, selenium, vitamin B6, and linoleic acid following plant enzyme supplements. Some dermatologists theorize that, since selenium is related to thyroid hormones, increased selenium absorption in some way affects thyroid hormones that allow the skin and hair to "normalize."

> Enzyme supplements are inexpensive, safe, and easy to administer in pill or, more commonly, powder form.

Enzymes rarely exert enough of an effect to serve as the sole therapy for pets with allergies. However, enzymes are one of the five types of supplements I recommend to improve the diets of all of my patients. Adding enzymes to the diet of allergic pets is particularly indicated to improve their overall nutritional status.

Doctors can prescribe pancreatic enzymes, microbial enzymes, or plant enzymes. To date, only the plant enzymes seem to help pets with allergies, so this is the type I recommend. The plant enzymes are active over a much wider pH range (pH 3 to 9) than pancreatic enzymes. Also, plants contain the enzyme cellulase, which dogs and cats do not produce in their bodies; that's why they can only digest some of the plant material in their diets. Supplements with enzyme products that contain cellulase in addition to the normal lipase, amylase, and proteases found in many supplements seem to be more advantageous to pets with medical problems such as atopic dermatitis. This may be due to the fact that cellulase liberates nutrients, such as zinc, bound in dietary fiber.

Enzyme supplements are inexpensive, safe, and easy to administer in pill or, more commonly, powder form. The powder is easily mixed with owner-prepared food or sprinkled on food fed in a dry form. Your doctor can help you decide which product is best for your pet's condition.

## Green Foods

Green foods, such as barley grass, spirulina, alfalfa, wheat grass, and algae, contain a variety of healthy nutrients. Supplementing with these products duplicates the grass that wild dogs ingest when they kill herbivorous prey animals.

Green foods contain large amounts of vitamins A, B1, B2, B6, C, and E; biotin; folic acid; choline; pantothenic acid; nicotinic acid; iron; chlorophyll; potassium; calcium; magnesium; manganese; zinc; proteins; and enzymes. Ingestion of these nutrients seeks to prevent and treat illnesses that may be induced by an imbalance of minerals, enzymes, and vitamins in processed foods.

Chlorophyll performs a number of healing services due to an anti-inflammatory effect. The enzymes contained in green foods aid in digestion and absorption of nutrients from the diet and also may assist in reducing inflammation in pets with allergic dermatitis. While I have not found green foods beneficial as a sole supplement for dogs with atopic dermatitis, they can be useful in combination with other supplements because they are anti-inflammatory. And, as is the case with enzymes, all pets can benefit from a diet supplemented with green foods.

## Oral Fatty Acids

Fats in the form of fatty acids have recently become a popular supplement among veterinarians, and not just those interested in holistic care. First suggested for use in treating allergies in pets, they are now advocated in cases of kidney disease, elevated cholesterol, and arthritis as well. Veterinarians are discovering that fatty acids can be valuable for a variety of conditions. So many doctors now use fatty acid supplements in treating atopic dermatitis in pets that, while I will discuss them in this chapter, they could almost be considered a conventional (although non-drug) therapy!

When I talk about using fatty acids, that doesn't mean adding some vegetable oil to the pet's diet to get a nice shiny coat. I'm referring to omega-3 and omega-6 fatty acids (omega-9 fatty acids have no known use in treating pets). Omega-3 fatty acids, eicosapentaenoic acid (EPA) and docosahexaenoic acid (DHA), are derived from fish oils of cold-water fish such as salmon and trout, and flaxseed. Omega-6 fatty acids, linoleic acid (LA) and gamma-linolenic acid (GLA), are derived from the oil of seeds such as evening primrose, black currant, and borage.

Since processed foods have increased omega-6 fatty acids and decreased omega-3 fatty acids, if your dog eats processed food, adding omega-3 supplements is probably a good idea. Adding large amounts of omega-3 fatty acids to a dog's diet favors the production of non-inflammatory eicosanoids, decreasing inflammation and itchiness in the pet with atopic dermatitis (see chapter 4, page 87). Eicosanoids produced from arachidonic acid are not the sole cause of the inflammation in pets with atopic dermatitis, however. For this reason, fatty acid therapy is rarely effective as the sole therapy, but is used with other therapies, often with other supplements, to achieve an additive effect.

**Obtaining Fatty Acids**   Fatty acids are supplied in a liquid "pump-bottle" form, and in a capsule form. Most pets take either form well. For dogs that are difficult to "pill," the liquid form is quite popular. Owners of dogs 20 pounds and under find the liquid form more cost effective than the large bottle of fatty acid capsules that we prescribe.

For owners who do not like giving their pets medication, or for pets who don't take the fatty acid supplements easily, it might be wise to try some of the medically formulated dog foods that contains the fatty acids. These are available from veterinarians, who often prescribe such food as an anti-inflammatory diet for pets with allergies. The main concern among holistic owners is that most of these "premium" diets are not natural, holistic products. Most of them contain fillers, by-products, and chemical preservatives and additives. A far better option is to feed a natural, processed food or better, a balanced homemade natural diet, and then supplement the diet with the recommended dosage of fatty acids.

If you are using packaged processed food as a source of fatty acids for your dog, be sure to check product labels carefully for the source of the fatty acid. Many processed diets supplemented with fatty acids use flaxseeds or flaxseed oil as the fatty acid supplement. While flaxseeds or flaxseed oil is not harmful to pets and does supply some essential omega-6 and omega-3 fatty acids, flaxseed oil is a source of alpha-linoleic acid (ALA), an omega-3 fatty acid that is ultimately converted to EPA and DHA. Many animals (probably including dogs) and some people cannot convert ALA to these other more active non-inflammatory omega-3 fatty acids, due to a deficiency of desaturase enzymes needed for the conversion. In one human study, flaxseed oil was ineffective in reducing symptoms or raising levels of EPA and DHA. Therefore, I do not recommend flaxseed oil as a fatty acid supplement for pets with atopic dermatitis. Instead, look for fish oil, which provides EPA and DHA. Flaxseed oil is often added to diets because fish oil produces a "fishy" smell that may be offensive to owners.

**Benefits of Fatty Acids**   A number of studies have documented the benefits of fatty acid supplements for allergic pets. These studies involved only a few of the many fatty acid supplements currently available, however. As is true with most nutritional supplements, the majority of supplement manufacturers have not paid for the expensive double-blind placebo-controlled studies so often required for definitive "proof" that the supplement actually works. This does not mean that only the few supplements tested are effective. Follow your doctor's advice when trying to choose a supplement for your pet. If one fatty acid supplement is ineffective, there are many others you can try.

In the literature, fatty acid supplements made from fish oil were effective in reducing symptoms of itching and inflammation in 11 to 27 percent of allergic dogs and over 50 percent of allergic cats. How well fatty acids work in an allergic pet depends upon a number of factors, including the product used, dosage, and the presence of other diseases that can contribute to itching. Many atopic pets also have flea allergies, bacterial skin infections, *Malassezia* yeast skin infections, and food hypersensitivity. Until these other concurrent problems are identified and treated properly, simply administering fatty acid supplements to a dog suspected of having only atopic dermatitis is unlikely to be effective.

In my practice, I have not found that the reported figures hold up. Few of my patients actually got better or even improved on fatty acid supplements without other complementary therapies. Therefore, while I discuss the research results with pet owners, I point out that in my practice I don't expect these results and therefore rarely use just fatty acids supplements as my main treatment. I don't know why I don't get these results, but I do know that any reported results are just guidelines and will vary among practice locations. In my part of the world, in Texas, year-round allergies are a problem for pets and their owners. I believe that atopic dermatitis is a harder disorder to control here than in other areas of the country. I understand that pets living along the Gulf Coast have a similar situation with flea allergy problems, unlike pets living in cooler, less humid climates.

While many veterinarians, including me, use fatty acids for a variety of medical problems, there is considerable debate about their use. One part of the debate concerns the dosage to use. Due to their anti-inflammatory effects, I routinely use large doses of fatty acids when treating atopic dermatitis in pets. Like most doctors, I recommend 2 to 4 times the label dose, as research in allergy treatment indicates that the label dose on most products is too low to exert an anti-inflammatory influence.

In people, research suggests that the effective dosage is from 1.4 to 2.8 grams of GLA per day, or 1.7 grams of EPA and 0.9 grams of DHA per day. It's hard for people to take that much using the supplements currently available because they come in a much lower dose. If this dosage is correct, translating this dosage to dogs (adjusting for weight) means a 50-pound dog would need to take 10 or more fatty acids capsules per day, depending upon the supplement.

Another concern is the correct fatty acid to use. Should we use just omega-3 fatty acids (EPA and DHA), or combine them with omega-6 fatty acids (GLA)? Is there an ideal ratio of omega-6 to omega-3 fatty acids? The ideal dietary ratio seems to be 5:1 of omega-6 to omega-3 fatty acids, although this is also debated. Whether or not this "ideal" dietary ratio is ideal for the treatment of allergies remains to be seen. According to one pet food manufacturer of premium (but not "natural") food, allergic pets eating their diet containing the "ideal" ratio of 5:1 omega-6 to omega-3 fatty acids showed improvement. Other dietary ratios failed to show the same improvement in allergic pets.

As with other supplements, the use of fatty acids often allows doctors to lower the dosages of drugs such as corticosteroids or antihistamines. As reported in the literature, some pets, especially those with mild clinical signs and whose owners are thorough with regular hypoallergenic shampooing and conditioning, respond quite favorable to using only fatty acid supplements, without the need for other therapies. As I mentioned, in my practice I haven't had good success with fatty acids alone.

Obviously, there are many questions regarding the use of fatty acid therapy as part of our treatment for allergic pets. While we have ample research showing that fatty acid supplements can be beneficial in pets with atopic dermatitis, more research is needed to determine the proper dosage and ratio of omega-6 and omega-3 fatty acids. Until we get definitive answers, you will need to work with your veterinarian (knowing the limitations of our current research) to determine the use of these supplements for your pet.

## Health Formula Blends

A number of products bear the claim that they are "health formulas." These products contain a variety of ingredients, including barley grass, wheat, rice, enzymes, fatty acids, vitamins, minerals, seaweed, and/or alfalfa. It isn't clear why these

## A CLOSER LOOK

Antioxidants function in the body to reduce oxidation. Oxidation is a chemical process that occurs within the body's cells. After oxidation occurs, certain by-products such as peroxides and free radicals accumulate. These cellular by-products are toxic to the cells and surrounding tissue. The body removes these by-products by producing additional chemicals called antioxidants that combat these oxidizing chemicals. In disease, excess oxidation can occur and the body's normal antioxidant abilities are overwhelmed. This is where supplying antioxidants can help. By giving your dog extra antioxidants, his body can neutralize the harmful by-products of cellular oxidation.

compounds often seem effective in the treatment of pets with atopic dermatitis. Obviously, they supply something that is missing from the diet, most likely antioxidants, vitamins, and minerals. Like fatty acid supplements, it may be that they in some way interfere with the production of pro-inflammatory compounds. Possibly they also supply nutrients for the cells of the skin to help heal and maintain "normal" skin. Since so many different blends are available, it is wise to discuss with your veterinarian whatever products you discover.

### Antioxidants

There are a number of antioxidants that may be beneficial as supplements for your allergic pet. The most common antioxidants are vitamins A, C, and E and the minerals selenium, manganese, and zinc. Other antioxidants, including superoxide dismutase, glutathione, cysteine, coenzyme Q10, ginkgo biloba, bilbery, grape seed extract, and pycnogenol, may also be helpful for pets with atopic dermatitis.

**Benefits of Antioxidants**    There is extensive research on the benefits of antioxidants for people. It is unknown if these same benefits of vitamin C and other vitamins and minerals occur in allergic pets. However, since there may be benefits, most holistic veterinarians recommend vitamin C and other antioxidant supplements for pets with atopic dermatitis.

In people with asthma, studies have detected decreased levels of vitamin C in the blood; it appears that asthmatics may have an increased need for vitamin C. Several studies showed improvements in asthmatics treated with daily doses of 1 to 2 grams of supplemental vitamin C. Research on humans has also found that vitamin C can increase the detoxification of histamine and prevent histamine secretion by white blood cells.

Vitamin E functions as an antioxidant and inhibits formation of leukotrienes, one class of chemicals that causes inflammation. The antioxidant vitamin A and related carotenes also decrease leukotriene formation.

Selenium, the mineral cofactor of vitamin E, may also be of benefit in allergic pets. As discussed in the section on enzymes, supplementing with selenium may be helpful in allergic pets due to its interaction with the enzyme glutathione peroxidase (see page 114).

Bioflavonoids, such as quercetin, are plant antioxidants. They can inhibit histamine release by mast cells and decrease leukotriene production. Quercetin has a sparing effect on vitamin C and stabilizes mast cell membranes,

# ORTHOMOLECULAR THERAPY FOR YOUR DOG*

A common orthomolecular therapy is to provide a combination of the antioxidants vitamin A, vitamin E, and selenium. Begin with a higher initial dosage and when you see a response in your dog such as decreased itching or redness, usually within 6 to 8 weeks, decrease dosage to maintenance levels.

## Initial Dosage

Vitamin A: 10,000 IU per day for small dogs, 20,000 IU for medium dogs, and 30,000 IU for large dogs.

Vitamin E: 800 IU for small dogs, 1,600 IU for medium dogs, and 2,400 IU for large dogs.

Selenium: 20 mcg for small dogs, 40 mcg for medium dogs, and 60 mcg for large dogs.

## Maintenance Dosage

Vitamin A: 1,250 IU for small dogs, 2,500 IU for medium dogs, and 5,000 IU for large dogs.

Vitamin E: 100 IU for small dogs, 200 IU for medium dogs, and 400 IU for large dogs.

Selenium: 2.5 mcg for small dogs, 5 mcg for medium dogs, and 7.5 mcg for large dogs.

*Due to potential toxicity with high doses of antioxidants, orthomolecular therapy should only be tried under veterinary supervision.

preventing their destruction and subsequent release of histamine and other chemicals that promote inflammation. Bioflavonoids, quercetin in particular, are found in grape seed, pine bark, green tea, and the herb ginkgo biloba.

Pycnogenol is often recommended as an antioxidant for patients with inflammatory disorders, including atopic dermatitis. Pycnogenol comes from the bark of pine trees native to southern France and is a mixture of bioflavonoids, also called proanthocyanidins. These bioflavonoids inhibit the prostaglandins and leukotrienes that cause inflammation and allergic responses. People taking pycnogenol often report feeling better and having more energy. Pets may experience similar benefits.

One source suggests that pycnogenol, like quercetin, seems to work by enhancing the effects of another antioxidant, vitamin C. Other research indicates that the bioflavonoids can work independently of other antioxidants; as is the case with many supplements, there probably is an additive effective in combining multiple antioxidants.

> Pycnogenol is often recommended as an antioxidant for patients with inflammatory disorders, including atopic dermatitis.

**Using Antioxidants for Atopic Dermatitis**    Orthomolecular therapy is the medical term for the treatment of disorders of pets using antioxidants. Several doctors report success with this therapy in dogs with atopic dermatitis. The idea behind using antioxidants for this condition is to optimize functioning of the immune system, prevent destruction of the cells of the skin, maximize adrenal gland function, and detoxify histamine. Discuss this option with your veterinarian. Orthomolecular therapy can be successful as part of a holistic approach to treating your dog's atopic dermatitis. The program should include feeding your dog a natural diet free of chemical preservatives and impurities, supplementing with fatty acids for overall good health, and obtaining a proper diagnosis of allergies.

In addition to other antioxidants such as vitamins A and E, many veterinarians give crystalline sodium ascorbate to bowel tolerance. Bowel tolerance is the dosage just below the level at which diarrhea (soft stool) is produced. When you see soft stool, lower the dosage to what you were giving before the soft stool occurred.

## Coenzyme Q10

Best known as a supplement for pets with heart disease, coenzyme Q10 is a vitamin-like substance resembling vitamin E. It exhibits antioxidant effects and works to reduce free radical damage caused by peroxidation of fatty acids. It plays an important role in the production of energy in the body's cells. Coenzyme Q10 appears to counter the inflammatory effects of histamine. While hard data is lacking, coenzyme Q10 may be beneficial in pets with allergic atopic dermatitis.

## Dimethylglycine (DMG)

DMG is a metabolic enhancer that is often used to improve performance and aid recovery from a variety of health problems. Studies in people and pets have shown that oral DMG supplements can improve the immune response. Due to this enhancement of the immune system and a potential anti-inflammatory effect, DMG is suggested by some as a therapy for a variety of disorders, including allergies in pets. More research is needed to determine the usefulness of DMG for atopic dermatitis in pets.

# Raw Foods and Glandular Products

Raw foods and glandular products are both used as therapies to treat diseases. Raw foods are processed whole foods that supply all of the biochemical components of the raw food, rather than just a single chemical fraction of a vitamin or mineral. Instead of giving a pet chemically produced "vitamin C" for allergies, a raw food product would supply vitamin C in its "natural" state. For example, a doctor might prescribe a whole (raw) food supplement made from carrots, broccoli, and wheat grass to provide the entire vitamin C complex rather than just administering chemically produced ascorbic acid, which is only a part of the entire vitamin C complex.

Glandular products are extracted from the glands of cattle, swine, or sheep, and concentrated by specific processes. These products have high biochemical activity designed to elicit specific nutritional or biochemical activity. For example, instead of giving a pet a chemically produced thyroid hormone, the doctor can prescribe a glandular extract from the thyroid gland of an animal.

### Benefits of Glandular Products

Proponents of glandular therapy in the veterinary field often recommend adrenal gland extracts for allergic pets to ensure proper immune function. This glandular product may work by boosting the levels of the adrenal gland hormone DHEA (dehydroepiandrosterone); research has found that some asthmatic people have decreased blood levels of DHEA.

Other studies on glandular products have shown there is an active accumulation of the injected cells or their constituents in the target tissues. There is a more rapid uptake of the corresponding injected cells in diseased organs than there is in normal organs, which may indicate an increased requirement by the diseased organ. Injected or implanted cells have tissue-specific effects on the corresponding tissues of the recipient. For example, thyroid cells given to animals with thyroid disease result in accelerated regeneration of the thyroid gland. Giving glandular products orally provides a longer-lived effect.

Finally, glandular preparations contain not only the active hormone substance, but a variety of substances with biologic activity, many of which have not been identified.

## Benefits of Raw Foods

With raw foods, the concept is simple: Why provide a chemical vitamin or mineral that represents only one fraction of the vitamin or mineral complex? Instead, feeding a whole-food product provides your pet with all of the nutrients found in that food.

Numerous studies demonstrate that the protection against disease is lost when synthetic vitamins are substituted for diets high in fresh fruits and vegetables. One older study, from 1942, showed that people suffering from scurvy, a vitamin C deficiency, healed when given either fresh vitamin C in the form of lemon juice or synthetic ascorbic acid, but that those getting the natural vitamin C in the lemon juice healed quicker than those receiving the synthetic. Another more recent study, reported in the *New England Journal of Medicine* (July 22, 1994), showed that synthetic antioxidants were not effective against recurrence of benign growths of the colon.

Yet, other studies have shown that diets high in natural vegetables and fruits did have protection against colon cancer.

Proponents of natural raw foods suggest that these findings are due to the presence of phytochemicals, the numerous compounds present in the whole plant. Using this theory, it is not just vitamin C or ascorbic acid (a component of vitamin C) that is helpful, but rather the entire plant that contains the entire complex molecule of vitamin C plus a number of other chemicals (many of which have yet to be identified).

> Feeding a whole-food product provides your pet with all of the nutrients found in that food.

One company has produced supplements for people that can also be prescribed for pets. Standard Process is a company founded on the belief of the superior value of vitamins and minerals in their whole raw-food states when compared to synthetic products. I recommend their whole food products Catalyn (a raw, natural vitamin-mineral supplement), Allerplex, Dermatrophin, and Livaplex (among others) for the treatment of atopic dermatitis.

While there is a lot of research showing that whole raw foods may be preferable to synthetic vitamins, many doctors who practice complementary therapies use synthetic vitamins with good success. Synthetic vitamins and minerals may be of use in pets, but their use should not take priority over the natural vitamins and minerals in raw food products.

My conclusion is: Feed pets a good wholesome diet free of by-products and preservatives; give them whole raw-food supplements for maintenance and disease treatment; and use synthetic vitamins as directed by your doctor if needed for additional treatment (for example, in conditions that may benefit from additional antioxidants, including atopic dermatitis, if the pet does not respond to raw food and glandular supplements). Whenever possible, due to the number of phytochemicals in raw foods, use these sources instead of chemically processed vitamins and minerals.

---

## CHAPTER SUMMARY

- Proper diagnosis is necessary before beginning any complementary therapy.

- Success for the allergic pet may be to make it comfortably itchy.

- Topical treatments including frequent shampooing and conditioning are essential in the care of the allergic pet.

- Proper diet and nutritional supplements provide your pet with a stronger immune system to fight secondary infections.

---

# ·6·

# Additional Complementary Therapies

I N ADDITION TO the treatments discussed so far, other complementary therapies may be of benefit to the pet with atopic dermatitis. These include herbs, acupuncture, and homeopathy.

## HERBAL TREATMENTS

THERE ARE A variety of herbs for treating the dog with atopic dermatitis. Doctors may prescribe the whole herb or just the active ingredient in the herb. Products vary as to whether they contain the whole herb or a part. By using only the active ingredient, you avoid the plant's toxins and substances that may make that ingredient less effective. By using only the active ingredient, however, you lose the substances that might act in conjunction with that ingredient. It is up to debate which is most beneficial.

A number of companies package herbs for the human and pet market, but standard quality controls such as those that exist for pharmaceuticals are lacking. Studies have shown that some products have more or less, and sometimes even none, of the active ingredient listed on the bottle! For this reason, purchase only products from high quality, reputable companies. In my own practice, I use only herbs from companies with whose quality control I feel most comfortable. The least expensive generic herbal supplements are likely to be of lowest quality and questionable value.

The study of herbal therapy can be divided into Western herbal therapy and traditional Chinese medicine (TCM), though the two use many of the same herbs.

## Western Herbal Therapy

With Western herbal therapy, a veterinarian makes a conventional diagnosis, as explained in chapter 4.

While herbal therapy can be effective in dogs with atopic dermatitis, more research is needed to find the "best" herb or herbal combination and the most useful dosages. There are few studies on the use of herbs for treating this condition in pets. Therefore, most of our information is extrapolated from human studies and clinical veterinary experience. Since so many other complementary therapies are quite effective in treating atopic dermatitis in pets, herbs are not used as frequently. Still, if you wish to use herbs for your allergic dog, it is important to be familiar with what is known about them.

You can administer herbs to your dog orally and/or topically, depending on the herb. For topical treatment, peppermint, chamomile, calendula, juniper, lavender, rose bark, or uva ursi herbal rinses can provide temporary relief from scratching. The following herbs may also be useful for atopic dermatitis:

**Alfalfa:** Alfalfa is a green food (see chapter 5, page 116) used as an anti-inflammatory, antioxidant, and a diuretic to cleanse the body.

**Aloe:** Apply aloe topically as a soothing rinse or topical cream or gel. The oatmeal shampoo and conditioner I use also contain aloe vera for its anti-inflammatory properties. Acemannan, an immune-stimulant glycoprotein found in aloe vera or the glycoprotein ambrotose, may also be helpful for pets with allergies and skin infections (see chapter 5, page 108). You should only use aloe externally on your dog; internal application exerts a strong laxative effect.

**Burdock root:** Burdock is used for its cleansing properties as well as diuretic effects. Burdock is a good liver tonic. It is also known for its benefits for any skin condition with oiliness, flakiness, and inflammation. Its diuretic action removes toxins and wastes from the body.

**Dandelion:** Useful for its ability to stimulate the liver, as a diuretic, and for its anti-inflammatory properties, dandelion is also a healthy green food providing a number of vitamins, minerals, and other nutrients to the pet.

**Echinacea:** Echinacea is used as an immune stimulant and as an antimicrobial herb. Since echinacea works best with a healthy immune system, accompanying its use with other herbs (such as goldenseal), nutritional supplements, and a proper diet boosts its effectiveness.

**Garlic:** Garlic is useful for atopic dermatitis because of its immune-stimulating, antibacterial, and antifungal properties. Garlic also contains chemicals that can reduce the production of inflammatory prostaglandins. Garlic and nutritional yeast are often used to control fleas, though scientific proof is lacking as to their effectiveness; some owners report positive results. Too much garlic can be toxic to pets, causing a condition called

Heinz body anemia. As a rule, I recommend following label directions for flea products. In feeding fresh garlic, I use 1 clove per 10 to 30 pounds of body weight per day.

**German chamomile:** Chamomile is an anti-inflammatory herb with antimicrobial properties and the ability to heal wounds. This makes it useful for dogs with atopic dermatitis and/or skin infections. A chamomile infusion can be applied topically to inflamed or infected skin. You can also apply the infusion topically to the eyes for pets with allergic conjunctivitis.

**Ginkgo biloba:** The bioflavonoids in ginkgo may inhibit histamine release by mast cells and decrease the production of chemicals, such as leukotrienes, that promote inflammation. Ginkgo also contains terpene molecules called ginkgolides. Ginkgolides antagonize platelet activating factor (PAF ). PAF, a chemical produced by the body, triggers allergies. Double-blind studies of asthmatic people showed that the anti-asthmatic effects of orally administered ginkgolides improved respiration. It required high doses of ginkgo extract to achieve this effect.

**Goldenseal:** Used as an antimicrobial and anti-inflammatory herb, goldenseal can be applied topically to open sores or inflamed skin. Pets with allergic conjunctivitis (runny eyes) may benefit from eyedrops made from goldenseal. Goldenseal should not be used in pregnant animals or in pets with low blood sugar, as goldenseal further lowers blood sugar. Long-term use of goldenseal may cause hypertension and overstimulate the liver.

**Licorice root:** Licorice root is known for its anti-inflammatory, antimicrobial, and immune-stimulating properties.

Its primary active ingredient is glycyrrhetinic acid, which behaves similarly to corticosteroids in that it inhibits inflammatory prostaglandins and leukotrienes. You can administer licorice root orally or topically. Since licorice has cortisone-like activity, similar side effects can be seen with long-term use, including increased thirst and urination and adrenal gland suppression. Licorice should not be used in pregnant or lactating animals. Since licorice can elevate blood sugar levels, caution is needed with diabetic pets.

**Nettle:** You can use nettle for its antihistamine properties and to support liver function in pets with chronic skin disorders. In people, one study showed that 58 percent of patients with allergic rhinitis (runny nose) found relief after taking nettle. Animals with plant allergies can be sensitive to nettle, so be sure to consult with a veterinarian before using this herb.

**Red clover:** Used as a tonic, diuretic, and blood cleanser, red clover contains a number of nutrients (including B and C vitamin complexes, and protein) that act synergistically to help pets with skin disorders. You can administer the herb internally, or externally as a rinse. The bioflavonoids in red clover purportedly help pets with cancer, including skin cancer. While definitive studies are lacking, it may be that these bioflavonoids also improve the immune system of pets with atopic dermatitis. You should not use red clover in pregnant or lactating animals, in pets with clotting disorders or hormonal disorders involving estrogen, or in pets sensitive to aspirin, as red clover contains small amounts of salicylic acid, the active ingredient in aspirin.

**Yellow dock:** A cleansing herb that stimulates liver function and evacuation of the bowels to remove wastes from the body, yellow dock is useful for chronic skin disorders that may be attributed to toxicity in the body. It is most commonly used on a short-term basis at the beginning of therapy to get a "quick cleansing." Excess yellow dock can lead to intestinal cramping, vomiting, and diarrhea; it should not be used during pregnancy.

## Traditional Chinese Medicine (TCM) Herbal Therapies

According to TCM, there is no one such entity as "allergies." Instead, TCM looks for deficiencies or excesses in various body systems. For example, a TCM doctor might prescribe one or more herbs to "relieve wind" in a dog who exhibits the signs of atopic dermatitis. According to TCM, excess wind in the body is a cause of itching. But another dog might have a different imbalance producing his itching and inflammation, and require a different set of herbs as treatment. The Western diagnosis is not important to the TCM doctor, as the herbal therapy is based on a different way of looking at the body. Once the doctor has determined the imbalance according to the TCM system, he or she may then prescribe a combination of herbs with Chinese names (often the herbs have Western names as well).

To my knowledge, there have been no reported controlled studies using Chinese herbal therapies in atopic pets. One study involving the use of Chinese herbs to treat the itching seen in 30 people infected with measles showed that seven people experienced significant improvement, 15 experienced moderate improvement, and 5 experienced slight improvement.

The following are herbs or herbal combinations used in TCM that may have application to a condition with the symptoms of atopic dermatitis:

**Angelica and rehmannia:** These tone the body and move blood to relieve rash and itching by extinguishing wind.

**Dictamnus:** This herb has antifungal action and relieves fire toxicity (excess heat is one of the imbalances TCM identifies).

**Ganoderma, ginseng, rehmannia, licorice, bupleurum, scute, *zizyphi fructus* (jujube), and sophora:** These are among the more common herbs containing plant steroids that can mimic the action of synthetic corticosteroids. Plant steroids usually have milder actions with minimal side effects compared to synthetic steroidal drugs.

**Gardenia:** An herb to clear heat, it reduces inflammation and redness, and also has good antibiotic effects.

**Licorice:** This root is used in TCM and Western herbal therapy. In TCM, it is used to harmonize the body and nourish tendons and muscles.

**Moutan, arctium, and lithospermum:** These herbs cool and detoxify the blood to decrease itching. Arctium also has good antibiotic effects.

**Schizonepeta, cicada, and siler:** All are used to relieve wind.

**Sophora, clematis, and kochia:** These herbs are used to drain dampness and relieve weepy skin lesions.

**Tribulus and anemarrhena:** These herbs can decrease itching and inflammation.

# USING HERBAL TREATMENTS

Herbs are most often used in powder, capsule, and tincture (concentrated liquid) form. Many products made for humans can be used by pets. Unfortunately, the correct dosage for pets has not been determined for many herbs. We have to rely on clinical experience and extrapolation from human data. The following guidelines serve as a starting point for herbal therapy for dogs:

## Western Herbs

1 500-mg capsule for every 25 pounds of body weight, given 2
   to 3 times daily

0.5 to 1.5 teaspoons of powder for every 25 pounds of body
   weight, given 2 to 3 times daily

5 to10 drops for every 10 pounds of body weight, given 2 to 3
   times daily

## Chinese Herbs

1 gram concentrated herbs for every 20 pounds of body weight,
   given 2 to 3 times daily

4 grams fresh herbs for every 20 pounds of body weight, given 2
   to 3 times daily

Both Chinese and Western herbal therapies can be useful in treating the atopic pet. It is important to try different herbs or combinations in order to match the correct therapy with the pet. While most pets can be successfully treated with other therapies without the use of herbs, some owners prefer herbal medicine, and some cases require a trial with herbs if they do not respond to other therapies.

# ACUPUNCTURE

ACUPUNCTURE CAN BE very effective in the treatment of the atopic dog. It is used both to treat the condition and as a general stimulant of the pet's immune system. In particular, electroacupuncture (see page 141), compared to traditional needle acupuncture, demonstrates great anti-inflammatory effects at the cellular level in pets with allergies. Remember, as allergens interact with antibodies located on mast cells found in the skin, the mast cells "explode," releasing a variety of chemical compounds from granules located within the mast cells. Acupuncture can counteract the effects of these chemicals. For example, acupuncture suppresses the leakiness of blood vessels caused by histamine release from mast cells. Decreased fluid from the blood vessels decreases inflammation and decreases itchiness in allergic pets.

> It is important to try different herbs or combinations in order to match the correct therapy with the pet.

I examined Bronwyn, a 3-year-old female Boxer with chronic skin infections, which a previous veterinarian had told the owner were probably due to atopic dermatitis. The infections seemed to be concentrated on the neck and mammary glands. I ordered a skin biopsy and skin culture, and referred the owner to a local allergist for skin testing. The results of testing indicated a skin infection secondary to atopic dermatitis. Bronwyn responded quite well to antibiotics, but would relapse shortly after the course of antibiotics ended. Despite antigen injections and nutritional supplements, she continued to need antibiotics to maintain normal skin. Antibiotics to treat skin infections are expensive, and long-term use is not especially good for pets.

Due to the owner's concerns over the cost and the shortening of her dog's life, she elected to try acupuncture to stimulate Bronwyn's immune system. I chose acupuncture points based upon our desire to stimulate the immune system; points were also chosen that were known to be effective in pets with atopic dermatitis. The points we used were LI-11, ST-36, SP-6, SP-10, and GV-14. After four treatments (2 per week, 15 minutes per treatment) with needle acupuncture, the skin was healed. Bronwyn has remained free of skin infections, with acupuncture treatments given every 1 to 3 weeks as needed. Her owner has not had to give Bronwyn antibiotics for several months now.

## Understanding Acupuncture

In traditional acupuncture, the acupuncturist inserts tiny painless needles at various points on the pet's body. The insertion is shallow and does not draw blood. The points correspond to areas of the body that contain nerves and blood vessels. By stimulating these points, many doctors theorize that acupuncture stimulates the release of various chemicals (endorphins and enkephalins) in the body. These chemicals, through inhibition of pain, stimulation of the immune system, and alterations in blood vessels, cause a decrease in the clinical signs.

Other forms of acupuncture involve laser therapy (using a laser to stimulate the chosen points); aquapuncture, in which tiny amounts of vitamins are injected at the acupuncture site for a more prolonged effect; and electroacupuncture, in which a small amount of electricity painlessly stimulates the acupuncture site for a more intense healing effect.

As a rule, acupuncture compares quite favorably with conventional therapies. Acupuncture can succeed where conventional medicine fails, as when conventional therapy is ineffective or potentially harmful, as in long-term therapy with drugs like corticosteroids. Although surgery is not an issue for allergies, acupuncture can be so effective that a pet receiving treatments may be able to avoid back surgery for intervertebral disk disease or hip replacement surgery in the case of severe hip dysplasia. Discuss this option with your holistic veterinarian.

Side effects from acupuncture are rare. Accidental puncture of a vital organ can occur. Infection can occur at the site of needle insertion. Occasionally, the needle can break and surgery may be needed to remove it. In some animals, signs may worsen for a few days before they improve. This is called a healing crisis and is often a sign that the body is getting rid of toxins.

Many owners worry that acupuncture is painful and that their pets will suffer. Acupuncture is normally painless. Remember, the needles are inserted quite shallowly. Occasionally, the animal may experience some sensation as the needle passes through the skin, but once the needle is in place, it is painless. Most animals relax and some become sleepy. Fractious animals may require mild sedation for treatment.

## Using Acupuncture

You should have a proper diagnosis before starting any treatment for allergies, including acupuncture. Only veterinarians can make a proper diagnosis for your dog and prescribe the correct course of therapy. Make sure the person performing acupuncture is a veterinarian experienced with this form of therapy.

Since starting acupuncture in my practice, I have become aware of and concerned by something that has caught me by surprise. Many of the pets I have seen for acupuncture consultation for various problems did not in fact have the problems for which I was consulted. Some of these pets had more serious problems, leading me to wonder how many pets are mistreated because they have not gotten an accurate diagnosis. Even when an animal has a condition that cannot be treated, it deserves a proper diagnosis to help it live a decent quality of life. For therapies to be effective, the doctor must understand what is going on in the pet's body.

> The acupuncture points used on pets with atopic dermatitis are those that strengthen the immune system and relieve itching and inflammation.

Many owners seem surprised that I stress this. It seems that these owners just want me to grab some needles and start treatment! But where do I place the needles? Will acupuncture help their pet? I can't answer these questions without a proper diagnosis.

The number of acupuncture treatments that a pet will require varies from pet to pet. Usually, owners are asked to commit to 8 treatments over 2 to 3 weeks to assess if acupuncture will work. On average, treatments last from 15 to 30 minutes for needle acupuncture, and 5 to 10 minutes for aquapuncture or electroacupuncture. If the pet improves, acupuncture is then performed as needed, depending on the pet's signs.

The acupuncture points used on pets with atopic dermatitis are those that strengthen the immune system and relieve itching and inflammation. Alternatively, the acupuncturist can use points to treat the condition as identified according to traditional Chinese medicine. Thus, the condition of a dog with atopic dermatitis may be wind-heat or damp-heat lodging in the skin. The acupuncturist then selects the appropriate points to treat these diagnoses.

# HOMEOPATHY

HOMEOPATHY, A SYSTEM of medical practice developed by Dr. Samuel Hahnemann in 1790, is the science of "like curing like." With conventional medicine, drugs are used to reduce symptoms or allow the body to cure the disease. Homeopathy uses the energy of dilute solutions to help the body heal.

Homeopathy is based on the belief that the same substances that cause a disease can, in a diluted form, cure the disease. The more dilute the homeopathic compound, the stronger it is in the treatment of the disorder.

To those who are hearing about homeopathy for the first time, I know this concept sounds quite strange. As a doctor trained in conventional medicine, I too was overwhelmed when I first heard about the concept of "like curing like." In homeopathic compounds, there is often no trace of the original ingredient. It may seem that all we're giving the pet is water and alcohol, which are the carriers for the original compound. And we certainly know that pets can't get better drinking water and alcohol.

Yet many do get better. While it's not 100 percent effective in every pet, homeopathic remedies do work. The idea is that even though the original substance may be gone because of multiple dilutions, the energy these compounds released when prepared stays in the solution and helps the pet heal.

Skeptics may point to a placebo effect. Certainly placebo effects are powerful in human medicine. You want to get better, you want the treatment to work, so it works. However, the placebo effect is all but impossible to reproduce or observe in pets. You can't tell your dog that the homeopathic remedy he's taking will make him stop itching, so he just decides to stop scratching! Either the treatment works or it fails.

> While it's not 100 percent effective in every pet, homeopathic remedies do work.

You must be open-minded and have a lot of faith when attempting homeopathic treatment for the first time. Often, pet owners think that homeopathy sounds bizarre and farfetched, so it is their treatment of last resort. Only after seeing side effects from drugs and going through all the other options will some owners consent to homeopathy. I understand. I've been there, too. When I first started learning about homeopathy, I thought it sounded too good to be true, and certainly it didn't make any sense from a Western scientific perspective. Yet after trying it a few times and seeing some impressive results, I became convinced that for some pets, homeopathy is a viable alternative or supplement to conventional treatment.

One of the good things about homeopathy is that it is virtually devoid of side effects. The substances are usually so dilute as not to cause any harm.

### Effectiveness of Homeopathy

Many of the pet owners who bring their animals to me swear that homeopathic remedies prescribed by their doctors have helped them in their own illnesses. I have seen a number of pets improve with homeopathy as well. As with any therapy, however, there are those cases for which no treatment is effective. Additionally, I rarely practice "pure" homeopathy, which means using only one or two homeopathic remedies as the treatment. I prescribe a number of therapies in addition to homeopathic remedies for my patients since these pets have chronic, often severe conditions. When they respond, it is impossible to say which particular therapy was effective. In many cases, there is probably a positive effect from the combination of treatments.

Some studies have shown positive effects in patients treated with homeopathic remedies when compared to placebos.

In *Dr. Rosenfeld's Guide to Alternative Medicine*, author Isadore Rosenfeld, M.D., quotes a study reported in the medical journal *The Lancet* that showed that asthmatics taking homeopathic remedies had a 30 to 40 percent improvement in their breathing when compared to those patients taking placebos. Another double-blind study showed that patients with hay fever who took homeopathic remedies required only half the dosage of antihistamines needed by patients taking placebos. Other studies quoted in his book showed no difference in patients taking homeopathic remedies when compared to patients taking placebos.

Dr. Rosenfeld's conclusion, which I agree with, is that homeopathy can help some patients, but more research is needed to understand the usefulness of homeopathy in treating allergic dogs.

## Using Homeopathy

Since many homeopathic remedies are available for purchase over-the-counter (OTC), which means without prescription. You might be tempted to skip a visit to the veterinarian and try using homeopathy on your own. Before trying any of these therapies on your pet, do see a holistic veterinarian and get a diagnosis. There is no one right remedy, and a thorough examination, history, and laboratory tests must be performed to assist the homeopathic veterinarian in selecting the correct remedy or remedies.

I recommend prompt and correct diagnosis, and using OTC homeopathic remedies only for the most minor clinical signs, such as mild itching and sneezing. If your dog (with even minor signs) does not improve in 2 to 3 days of treatment with an OTC remedy, take him to your veterinarian for proper evaluation of his condition.

Many OTC remedies are combination remedies rather than a single one. As mentioned above, traditional homeopathy identifies the one or two remedies that most closely match your pet's constitution and symptoms.

OTC remedies are the least dilute and least potent remedies that can be used to treat your pet. While not harmful, the more powerful prescription remedies available through your doctor are more likely to be effective.

Most important, all pets with itching are not necessarily allergic. Failing to seek medical help and trying home remedies can delay necessary treatment of a more serious condition. While homeopathy can be helpful, you should only treat pets with homeopathic remedies under a doctor's supervision!

Since I believe in treating the pet, not just the disease, I never use homeopathic remedies without also making sure the dog has a proper diet and giving him nutritional supplements.

Some homeopathic remedies that can help the atopic dog include:

*Arsenicum album:* This popular homeopathic remedy is used for pets with dry, scaly skin and harsh, dry coats.

*Antimonium crudum:* This is often recommended when the skin lesions are more pronounced on the back, neck, and limbs. The lesions often begin as red papules that ooze a yellow secretion and then form scabs.

*Cortisone:* As with traditional corticosteroids, homeopathic cortisone can be prescribed when itching and inflammation occurs. Unlike conventional steroids, there are no harmful side effects with homeopathic cortisone.

*Hepar sulphuris:* Prescribed for any condition involving pus, this remedy can help dry up the pus-filled pustules in a skin disorder complicated by secondary bacterial infection.

*Hypericum:* Often recommended for nerve injuries, this remedy is useful for pets whose allergies and skin conditions worsen with exposure to sunlight.

*Lycopodium:* This remedy is used when the skin condition involves hair loss. Homeopathic veterinarians prescribe this remedy to help stimulate the growth of hair, if the disease has not progressed so far that the hair follicles have been permanently damaged.

***Rhus toxicodendron:*** This is a good general remedy for a variety of disorders. Pets whose skin symptoms are aggravated by dampness and who seem stiff when moving, but then feel better after a few minutes of movement often respond to this remedy. It is also prescribed for skin that is red and itchy, and shows papules and pustules.

***Staphylococcinum:*** A homeopathic bacterial nosode, this product functions as a homeopathic "vaccine," targeting the most common bacterial invader of your pet's diseased skin. This remedy is used with other homeopathic remedies for pets with secondary bacterial infections, and can be tried in cases of mild infection, before or with antibiotics.

***Sulphur:*** This is one of the most commonly prescribed homeopathic remedies for pets with skin disorders, including atopic dermatitis. It is used to treat red and itchy skin that worsens with heat. It is also indicated for pets with secondary infections or fleabites, as indicated by the presence of papules or pustules. Many homeopathic doctors prescribe sulphur in conjunction with other more specific skin remedies to enhance their actions.

***Thuja:*** Not specifically for skin diseases (other than warts), this remedy is often recommended as an "antidote" for immune systems overwhelmed by repeated and often unnecessary vaccinations. Many holistic doctors are concerned about vaccinations, often suggest a cleansing remedy such as *Thuja* to decrease any contribution of vaccinations to the skin and other disorders.

To achieve success with any complementary or conventional therapy, your dog needs a solid foundation of good health, which can only be built with a proper diet. The next chapter discusses a good general diet, as well as the special dietary needs of the allergic dog.

## CHAPTER SUMMARY

- Herbal therapy, both Western and traditional Chinese medicine, can benefit the allergic pet.

- You can administer herbs to your dog internally, or externally as a rinse or topical treatment.

- Acupuncture and homeopathy are additional approaches for treating atopic dermatitis.

# ·7·

# Diet and Allergic Dermatitis

ONE OF THE most important factors you can control with regard to your dog's health care is diet. Your pet eats once if not more often each day, and you and you alone control what goes into his mouth.

Since diet directly affects pets and the diseases they acquire, including atopic (allergic) dermatitis, I like to spend a little time in each book in THE NATURAL VET™ series discussing diet. Here, I'll talk about some of the basics of nutrition first, then about how to find or prepare the most natural, healthiest diet for your pet. Finally, I'll show you some specific recommendations on altering diet to improve the health of your allergic dog.

To begin, here are some important questions I'd like you to ponder:

- Are you feeding your dog a healthy diet, with natural nutritional supplements?

- Are you instead feeding whatever food was on sale at your local pet store or grocery store?

- Is there any difference between the various diets on the market?

- Are premium diets really worth their cost?

It is important to consider how diet can affect the dog with atopic dermatitis. While most veterinarians and pet owners neglect the contribution diet makes to a pet's health, holistic doctors and holistic-minded owners know that proper diet and nutritional supplements can have a positive effect on the dog with atopic dermatitis. In fact, proper diet is the foundation of every holistic health plan.

# A Proper Diet

Just what constitutes the "best" or most appropriate diet for a dog is quite a controversial topic, and there are just as many opinions as there are veterinarians. Many pet owners and doctors express very firm views when asked these questions. Often their opinions are based more on emotion than on any objective medical facts. Part of the problem is that, even if someone goes looking for those facts, they can be difficult to find.

I'm going to ask you to put aside for a moment any preconceived ideas you might have when it comes to this subject. In choosing the most holistic option, keeping an open mind is essential. When you have learned about the various approaches to diet, you can form your own opinion, based upon your circumstances.

As a rule, you need to be concerned about the amount of food your dog eats as well as the general quality and specific nutritional content of that food. All dog food is not the same. You have a choice about the type of food you give your pet. Your choices fall into the general categories of processed food or natural-style food. Natural-style foods can be packaged or homemade. If you decide to prepare your dog's food at home, as many holistic pet owners do, you will need to decide if it should be raw or cooked. No matter what type of diet you choose, it must meet these five requirements:

1. The diet must include the proper amount and balance of essential nutrients required by your dog.
2. The ingredients must be of high nutritional quality so that your dog can effectively digest, absorb, and utilize the dietary nutrients.
3. The food should be palatable so your dog will eat it.
4. The food should contain no "fillers," such as animal or plant by-products. If by-products are included, as in the case of some prescription-type diets for sick pets, the food should contain the least amount of by-products.
5. There should be no artificial colors, flavors, chemical preservatives, or additives in your dog's diet, if possible.

## PACKAGED DOG FOOD

PROCESSED DOG FOODS have been around for 40 to 50 years. Prior to the introduction of processed dog food, our pets ate what we ate (or ate the leftovers of what we ate). Many holistic pet owners feel that pets fared much better then. I have heard some people go so far as to claim that atopic dermatitis is a disease of processed food, meaning that pets fed natural diets do not suffer from allergies. While I disagree, since I see pets who are eating good diets but are afflicted with allergies, I do agree that diseases including allergies would be less common if we fed our pets better diets.

Manufacturers developed processed dog food for the convenience of pet owners. Just as processed foods for humans save people a lot of time in food preparation, so too do processed pet foods make feeding your dog simple, easy, and quick. There is no question that it takes at least some time to properly prepare homemade food. On the other hand, it is quite convenient and fast to simply open a can or scoop a cup of food from a bag and feed the pet.

> Just as processed foods for humans save people a lot of time in food preparation, so too do processed pet foods make feeding your dog simple, easy, and quick.

Manufacturers also introduced processed dog food to address the concern of pet owners that their dogs get a nutritious diet. Pet owners began to see that simply tossing their dogs some scraps wasn't going to give them a complete, balanced diet.

Prior to our scientific understanding of nutrition, both people and pets suffered from diseases resulting from dietary imbalances. For example, people who didn't eat fruits or vegetables got scurvy as a result of vitamin C deficiency. Pets fed mainly meat developed nutritional osteodystrophy (nutritional secondary hyperparathyroidism) as a result of calcium deficiency. Cats fed only fish developed thiamine deficiency and steatitis, an inflammation of body fat.

By learning about the nutritional needs of pets and formulating balanced diets, these nutritional problems can be avoided. While many of the nutritional diseases seen prior to the introduction of processed food have all but been eliminated, there is no question that processed foods, specifically those of low nutritional quality and loaded with by-products and chemicals, may actually be contributing to a whole new set of problems.

When I think of packaged dog food, I think of three categories: the least expensive generic processed dog food, the more expensive premium dog food, and the most expensive natural-style dog food.

Generic dog food is the least expensive, but also the least healthy for your pet. Manufacturers use the cheapest ingredients possible. These are the foods that contain ingredients such as animal and plant by-products. Generic food is also more likely to contain numerous preservatives and additives. By reading the label, you can easily discern how unhealthy these foods are for your dog. Most generic foods are not tested on pets in feeding trials, but instead meet arbitrary nutritional "standards." Do not feed your dog generic dog food, as health problems due to nutritional deficiencies can result.

Premium dog foods are available at many pet stores and veterinary hospitals. They usually have higher quality ingredients than the generic foods. You must read the label on these foods, however. Many contain products from plants sprayed with pesticides and animals given hormones and chemical-laden feed. While some premium dog food can be an acceptable choice when properly combined with natural supplements, this type of food is not my first choice if the more natural-style diets are available. With many other brands, however, the only thing premium about them is the price. Reading the label can help you identify which foods to avoid.

The price of pet food is often a good indicator of quality. It would be impossible for a company that sells a generic

# READ THE LABEL!!!

Reading and understanding pet food labels is critical when choosing a packaged food. The label can help you determine the difference between the classes of packaged food and what's really behind the ingredients as they are listed. Many pet owners tell me that the label on their brand says the food is nutritionally complete, so therefore it must be good. This is not necessarily true. Here are a few tips on reading the labels on pet food.

1. Ingredient list: Ingredients are usually listed on packaged food labels in descending order from highest concentration to lowest. The first ingredient makes up the largest amount by weight of the ingredients. A meat-based source of protein should be among the first two or three ingredients in the food.

2. Guaranteed analysis: This states the minimum levels of nutrients in the food. A food with a minimum level of 5 percent protein means that the food has at least 5 percent protein; it may have a lot more, possibly even too much! Also, there is no guarantee that this protein is a good-quality protein. Chicken feathers have at least 5 percent protein, but I promise you that your pet won't get any nutrients from this protein source!

3. Digestibility: Poultry meal is a common protein source in pet food, but the digestibility of poultry meal varies from poor to excellent. Reputable manufacturers use higher quality ingre-

dients; the quality of the ingredient is reflected in the cost of the food. Stay away from cheaper generic brands with low digestibility.

4. Nutritional adequacy: Many products state that the food has been "formulated to meet the nutrition levels established by the AAFCO." (AAFCO is the American Association of Feed Control Officials.) Unfortunately, this just guarantees that the food meets a mathematical minimum. Your pet may not be able to digest or absorb anything in it, because the food never had to go through feeding trials to assess palatability and digestibility, and show if the animals in the trials grew or showed signs of malnutrition. The statement "animal feeding tests using AAFCO procedures substantiate that this food provides complete and balanced nutrition" means the food was fed to at least some pets for extended periods of time without detection of nutritional problems. The better, more expensive brands use this designation after conducting costly feeding trials. Read these labels carefully too, however. Just because the food passed feeding trials does not mean it does not contain chemical, additives, and fillers. There are many good, natural foods that have not undergone feeding trials. Work with your doctor to determine which food is best for your allergic dog.

brand of dog food at $9.95 for a 40-pound bag to use quality protein and grain in its food. The cost of purchasing quality ingredients would be much higher than the selling price.

## Natural-Style Packaged Dog Food

Natural-style dog foods are the top-of-the-line in packaged dog foods. They contain no artificial colors or flavors, and use natural rather than chemical preservatives. Instead of by-products, they use more expensive ingredients; depending upon the brand, these ingredients are from animals and plants raised organically without hormones or chemicals. Due to this insistence on quality and natural health, these foods are the best ones (and many would argue the only prepared foods) to feed your pet if you choose not to prepare a homemade diet.

Usually, because of the high quality of their ingredients, they are the most expensive packaged dog food. You really do get what you pay for when it comes to dog food. In my opinion, the health benefits of decreased disease and the resulting savings in veterinary care more than compensate for the increased price of the food. Dog food brands in this category include Wysong, Solid Gold, and Innova. The natural-style dog foods differ from most other packaged dog foods in the following ways:

- Natural-style dog food uses only human-grade, high-quality ingredients. Other prepared dog food may use by-products of foods processed for humans, but the by-products have been declared "unfit" for human consumption.

- Natural-style dog food uses foods, especially grains, in their whole state rather than only including a part. For example, this type of food contains whole rice rather than rice flour.

- Natural-style dog food uses no artificial colors, additives, chemicals, or preservatives.

- Natural-style dog food is formulated for optimum nutrition.

## What's Really in Pet Food

The information in this section is adapted from the copyrighted material on the Web site of the Animal Protection Institute (www.api4animals.com) and used with permission.

Most consumers are unaware that the pet food industry is an extension of the human food industry, also known as the agriculture industry. Pet food provides a place for slaughterhouse waste and grains considered "unfit for human consumption" to be turned into profit. This waste includes cow tongues, esophagi, and possibly diseased and cancerous meat. The "whole grains" used have had the starch removed and the oil extracted (usually by chemical processing) for vegetable oil; or they are the hulls and other remnants from the milling process. If whole grains are used, they may have been deemed unfit for human consumption because of mold, contaminants, or poor storage practices.

> Those companies devoted to producing natural, holistic food are more likely to use fresher, human-grade ingredients that are better for your pet.

There are many different brands of pet food available in this country. While many of the foods on the market are virtually the same, containing ingredients as described above, not all of the pet food manufacturing companies use these poor quality and potentially dangerous ingredients. Those companies devoted to producing natural, holistic food are more likely to use fresher, human-grade ingredients that are better for your pet.

There are both bad and good sources of ingredients commonly listed on commercial pet food labels. Here are the common ingredients and what you should know about where they come from.

**Protein:** The proteins in processed foods come from a variety of sources. There is a large amount of confusion among pet owners when they read terms like chicken, chicken meal, and chicken by-product meal. Here is how these terms are defined by AAFCO (American Association of Feed Control Officials).

- **Chicken:** The clean combination of flesh and skin, with or without the accompanying bone, derived from the parts or whole carcasses of chickens, exclusive of feather, heads, feet, and entrails.

- **Chicken meal:** The dry rendered product from a combination of flesh and skin, with or without accompanying bone, derived from the parts or whole carcasses of chickens, exclusive of feather, heads, feet, and entrails.

- **Chicken (or poultry) by-product meal:** Consists of the ground, rendered, clean parts of slaughtered chicken (or poultry) such as necks, feet, undeveloped eggs, intestines, exclusive of feathers, except in such amounts as occur in good rendering practices.

**By-products:** When animals are slaughtered, the choice cuts, such as lean muscle tissue, are trimmed away from the carcass for human consumption. Whatever remains of the carcass (bones, blood, pus, intestines, ligaments, and almost all the other parts not generally consumed by humans) is used in pet food. Such ingredients are listed on pet food labels as meat, poultry, or fish by-products, without detailing the actual contents. Many of these by-products are indigestible and provide a poor source of nutrition for dogs. The amount of nutrition found in the by-products of the meat, poultry, and fishing industries varies from vat to vat of dog food.

Some holistic veterinarians claim that feeding slaughterhouse wastes to animals increases their risk of getting cancer and other degenerative diseases. While this remains to be proven, there is no doubt that feeding these by-products provides little nutrition and may actually cause various diseases.

**Fat:** If you have ever noticed a pungent odor when you open a new bag of pet food, you are smelling refined animal fat, kitchen grease, and other oils too rancid for human consumption or deemed otherwise inedible.

Restaurant grease has become a major component of feed-grade animal fat over the last 15 years. This grease is usually kept outside for weeks, exposed to extreme temperatures with no regard for its future use. Rendering companies pick up this rancid grease and mix the different types of fat together, stabilize them with powerful antioxidants to retard further spoilage, and then sell the blended products to pet food companies.

These fats are sprayed directly onto dried kibble or extruded pet food pellets to make an otherwise bland or distasteful product palatable. The fat also acts as a binding agent to which manufacturers add other flavor enhancers. Pet food scientists have discovered that animals love the taste of these sprayed fats.

**Carbohydrates and grain products:** The amount of grain products used in pet food has risen over the last decade. The availability of nutrients in grain products is dependent upon the digestibility of the grain. The amount and type of a carbohydrate in pet food determine the amount of nutrient value the animal actually gets. Dogs (and cats) can almost completely absorb carbohydrates from some grains while up to 20 percent of other grains can escape digestion. A carbohydrate that escapes digestion is of little nutritional value due to bacteria in the colon that ferment carbohydrates. Some ingredients, such as peanut hulls, are used strictly for "filler" and have no nutritional value at all!

Many pet food companies use a technique called splitting to hide the fact that products with less nutritive value actually make up the bulk of the diet. For example, a pet food might list chicken, ground yellow corn, and corn gluten meal. The latter two ingredients are both corn-based products, basically the same ingredient. By listing them separately, it appears there is less corn than chicken in the product, even though the combined weight of the corn ingredients outweighs the chicken and should therefore be listed first on the label.

**Flavorings:** Garlic and onion are flavorings often added to processed foods. In the case of natural-style diets, garlic is often added for its purported medicinal properties as an antibacterial, anticancer, immune-stimulating element. At the dosages listed, the concentration of garlic is unlikely to be toxic and may be helpful to the pet. Onions, on the other hand, are potentially more toxic, especially for cats who can develop severe anemia from eating them. I do not recommend including onions in food for dogs or cats.

**Additives and preservatives:** Owners who desire to feed their pets a natural, chemical-free diet should be concerned about additives and preservatives. Many additives are added to commercial pet foods to improve the stability, appearance, or odor of the food. Additives provide no nutritional value and are mainly used to make the food appealing to pet owners; they are, after all, the ones who buy it. Since pets are mostly color-blind, a dog doesn't care what color his food is. However, the owner may prefer to feed the dog food that is red like fresh raw meat rather than brown like old meat. The artificial coloring used in this case has no nutritive value.

Additives also include emulsifiers to prevent water and fat from separating and anti-caking chemicals to keep ingredients from binding together. Antimicrobials reduce spoilage Antioxidants are used as preservatives to pre-

> Some ingredients, such as peanut hulls, are used strictly for "filler" and have no nutritional value at all!

vent fat from turning rancid and to prolong the shelf life of the product. Preservatives are necessary ingredients in pet foods, but natural antioxidants like vitamin C and vitamin E are better than chemical products such as ethoxyquin (EQ), butylated hydroxyanisole (BHA), and butylated hydroxtoluene (BHT).

According to research by the Animal Protection Institute, two-thirds of pet foods contain preservatives added by the manufacturer. Of the remaining third, most include ingredients already stabilized by synthetic preservatives. For example, premixed vitamin additives that must be added to pet foods to replace the vitamins lost during the processing of the food can also contain preservatives. This means that your dog may actually eat food with a variety of preservatives that have been added at the rendering plant, at the manufacturing plant, and in the supplemental vitamins.

Just as many people are realizing the effects that the chemicals added to processed foods have on our bodies, holistic doctors and concerned pet owners are realizing what the chemicals in processed pet foods are doing to dogs. There are a number of chronic disorders, such as various cancers, immune diseases, arthritis, and allergies, that are blamed on the chemicals found in pet foods. Even though these chemicals in the low amounts in pet foods are regarded as safe, we have no firm data on whether or not they may be related to these chronic disorders.

> There are a number of chronic disorders, such as various cancers, immune diseases, arthritis, and allergies, that are blamed on the chemicals found in pet foods.

In some cases (as with ethoxyquin), the many years of use seem to suggest "safety," but there may be a toxic accumulation effect. In the last 40 years, the number of food additives has greatly increased. Of the many recognized food additives today, no toxicity information is available for 46 percent of them. Cancer-causing chemicals are sometimes permitted if they are used at levels considered safe. The risk of continued ingestion of these cancer-causing agents has not been studied and the buildup of these chemicals may be harmful.

# A CLOSER LOOK

Ethoxyquin (EQ), butylated hydroxyanisole (BHA), and butylated hydroxtoluene (BHT) are the chemical antioxidant preservatives most commonly used in processed food for animal consumption. While ethoxyquin use is worrisome among pet owners, 75 years of study conclude that the product appears to be safe when used at the low concentration of 0.015 percent. Additionally, research has shown that ethoxyquin can interfere with cancer induction by other chemicals (by binding carcinogenic chemicals and enzymes that convert harmless chemicals into those that can cause cancer).

Many holistic doctors, however, claim that ethoxyquin is a major cause of disease, skin problems, and infertility in dogs. As a result, many pet owners fear using ethoxyquin, so most of the better pet food manufacturers have stopped using it, along with BHA and BHT. They have replaced these chemical preservatives with natural antioxidants such as vitamins C and E. While BHA and BHT are also approved for use in people and animals at the recommended "safe" levels, most holistic pet owners prefer to avoid processed foods containing these chemicals as well.

The reason for the prevalence of the chemical preservatives is that they cost less than vitamins C and E. The cheaper generic dog foods are most likely to contain the less expensive chemical preservatives. Once again, read the label if you choose to give your dog processed food.

Whenever possible, the healthier alternative is to purchase natural-style dog food that does not contain chemicals or to prepare healthy homemade recipes. If you must feed your dog a processed food other than the natural-style, look for one that lists the least amount of chemical additives. This will reduce toxicity to your dog. With any kind of processed food, supplement with natural products such as brewers yeast, fatty acids, kelp, barley grass, cooked liver, enzyme products, and sprouted beans or seeds to help replace nutrients lost during processing.

# Homemade Diets

If you're willing to prepare food for your pet at home, know that most holistic doctors feel that a homemade diet is simply the best food for your pet. This section will teach you how to do just that.

Raw or cooked? As a pet owner, you may have heard a lot of arguments for or against feeding your dog raw food versus cooked food. Many owners feel that feeding a raw diet is the only way to offer a truly healthy diet, and that cooking destroys the nutritional value of the food.

Since this topic is so controversial, with little science to back up either side, I would like to address the key arguments made for and against feeding raw foods.

### The BARF Diet

The argument over raw versus cooked pet food really concerns what has become known as the BARF diet (also called the Billinghurst diet, after Dr. Ian Billinghurst, the doctor who came up with this concept). BARF is a humorous acronym for Bones And Raw Food. In this diet, the pet is fed raw bones, raw meat, raw vegetables, and a carbohydrate source such as rice. The concept is simple: since the wild relatives of our pets eat raw meat, that is what our pets should eat. Let's take an objective look at the main claims by proponents of this diet.

**Claim:** Pets should eat what their wild relatives eat.

**Consideration:** While it is true that their wild relatives eat raw, freshly killed foods, our dogs are not wild animals, but domestic ones. That doesn't mean we can't feed them a similar diet, only that we need to keep in mind that these are totally different groups of animals with different lifestyles, exercise patterns, and health concerns.

**Claim:** Raw meat is safe for our pets; wild animals suffer no ill effects from raw meat.

**Consideration:** Whether or not raw meat is safe is debatable, although most pet owners report no obvious health problems in pets fed raw meat. Conversely, many owners report healthier looking coats and skin, less itching, less arthritis, and general overall health improvement once pets are fed raw homemade diets. There are health concerns, such as parasites and bacterial contamination, when feeding raw meat. These are discussed at length further along in this discussion.

To say that wild animals suffer no ill effects from eating raw meat is ignorant and presupposes we know everything that happens to every wild animal. While most wild animals thrive on their diets (as would be expected), we also know that wild prey carry parasites, which are transmitted to wild animal predator relatives of our pets, and that any infected meat could certainly cause illness in a wild animal. Unfortunately, no studies that I am aware of have pursued this topic.

**Claim:** Animals are more "acidic" compared to people. That is why they don't get sick eating raw meat.

**Consideration:** I'm not sure what this statement means, or how someone could even measure a pet's "acidity." I assume that those who make this statement believe that the "acid" in the pet's body can detoxify anything bad in the diet. While it is true that wild animals have adapted to their diets, this in no way means that they are immune to problems associated with the diet. For example, if a wild animal were only able to eat the muscle meat on the prey, that animal would develop calcium deficiency as meat is low in calcium. If the meat were rancid and infected with bacteria, the animal could certainly develop food poisoning (as often happens with pets that get into and eat garbage). If an animal eats meat infected with parasites, the animal gets infected with the parasite. So this statement concerning acidity just doesn't hold up.

**Claim:** Raw meat is safe for our pets. Their systems are designed to handle any problems with meat.

**Consideration:** This all depends what is meant by "safe." Certainly raw meat from animals raised free of chemicals and hormones, and that isn't infected with bacteria or parasites, is safe. Owners who choose to feed raw meat must do all they can to ensure that this meat is "safe" and free from pesticide, chemical, and hormonal residues as well as parasite ova (eggs.) Proper handling of the meat is needed to ensure that it stays "safe" at home (most food poisoning results from improper handling at home rather than a problem with the actual source of the meat itself).

When pet owners say that animals can handle problems with raw meat, I assume they mean that the digestive tract and immune system of a pet (and of a wild animal) can eliminate any infections or parasites before they cause problems for the animal. While it is true that a healthy pet is less likely to succumb to an infection or develop disease when infected with parasites (although this depends upon the type of parasite and the number infecting the animal), raw meat can still make an animal sick. Following the guidelines in the next section for the safe use of raw meat will make this highly unlikely, however, and you may feel a raw diet is worth the risk.

What I find interesting is the recommendation that it is acceptable to feed raw meat, except for raw pork or raw wild game (venison, rabbit, etc.), to pets. The reason for this warning, which I agree with, by the way, is that these meats are more likely to harbor parasites than beef or lamb. However, this warning seems contradictory. If our pets "can handle" raw meat because of their "acidity" and their immune systems, why can't they handle the parasites present in any raw meat? In the wild, animals eat raw pork, venison, and a whole host of other meats that proponents of raw diets caution against us feeding to our pets. To me, this is an obvious discrepancy that discredits their argument about raw meat being totally safe for pets.

**Claim:** Feeding dogs bones is safe.

**Consideration:** Once again, we need to define "safe." Most pets eating raw bones do not die, develop impaction of the digestive tract, or experience any health problems.

Still, some do, as most veterinarians can attest. Some proponents state that only cooked bones, which are softer than raw uncooked bones, are likely to splinter and cause problems. Once again the choice about feeding bones is up to your discretion.

While it may seem that the evidence presented so far in this discussion suggests dogs should not eat raw meat or bones, that is not necessarily the case. We have no good studies comparing the health of pets eating raw versus cooked foods, nor do we have any studies comparing the safety of either diet. I can say that many of my clients feed raw meat and bones to their dogs and have not reported any problems. In fact, many of these pet owners feel that their pets are healthier, have shinier coats, shed less, and have fewer health problems such as itching and arthritis. Some proponents of a raw diet suggest that problems such as arthritis are due to processed foods and are not seen in animals fed raw food. While I do not totally agree with this assessment, I do agree that pets eating the best diet, combined with high-quality supplements, can maintain a healthier lifestyle than those eating highly processed foods containing by-products and chemical preservatives.

The choice is ultimately yours. Regardless of what you decide to feed your dog, it is important to properly supple-

> Some proponents of a raw diet suggest that problems such as arthritis are due to processed foods and are not seen in animals fed raw food.

ment his diet to prevent deficiencies and ensure maximum health. For a complete discussion of nutritional and other supplements, see chapter 5.

## Making Homemade Dog Food

To prepare natural, chemical-free food for your dog, begin by selecting the freshest ingredients. Ideally, the vegetables and meats should be from plants and animals raised without chemicals, hormones, or pesticides. Most homemade diets use beef or poultry as the main protein source. You can use lamb, venison, or rabbit, but I prefer to reserve these protein sources for pets that have medically confirmed food allergies. In terms of preparation, my approach is to cook any meat and the grains; vegetables can be raw or lightly cooked.

If you have decided to feed your dog raw food, there are certain measures you should take to minimize the risk to your dog. While veterinarians who are holistic purists often recommend feeding a dog raw food, and while many of these doctors have not had problems with food poisoning as a result of their recommendations, you would be wise to be concerned about the possibility of infection from raw meat. The bacteria of immediate concern are E. coli and Salmonella. The media regularly carry stories about human illness and death from both of these organisms. E. coli seems to be of most concern from beef, whereas Salmonella seems to occur mostly as a result of ingestion of poultry products (raw chicken, turkey, and eggs).

The following guidelines can reduce the likelihood of your dog getting a bacterial or parasitic infection from eating raw meat, but they are not foolproof.

1. Only feed chicken, turkey, lamb, or beef raw; it is best to cook rabbit, venison, wild game, and pork.

2. Cook ground meats (unless you grind them at home) to prevent cross-contamination with other foods at the local grocery or butcher shop.
3. Freeze all meats for at least one week prior to feeding.
4. Thoroughly wash all meat in clean water prior to feeding. Only prepare the amount that will be fed at that meal, and keep the remaining meat frozen.
5. At any sign of illness (as a result of feeding raw meat), take your dog to your veterinarian at once for evaluation.

Dietary deficiencies (mainly vitamins and minerals) are more common with a homemade diet. Careful attention to proper preparation is critical to prevent both nutritional deficiencies and excesses. You should add multivitamin/mineral preparations designed for puppies or adult dogs to the food you make. Some holistic practitioners also recommend the addition of colloidal minerals, which purportedly are a better vehicle for delivery of minerals to the pet, although this claim is unsubstantiated. Calcium can be added in the form of bonemeal or calcium tablets (gluconate, carbonate, or the lactate forms are acceptable); natural calcium supplements (such as those made by Standard Process) are preferable to synthetic substitutes.

# DIETARY RECOMMENDATIONS FOR ALLERGIC DOGS

NOW THAT YOU understand a bit more about feeding your dog well for good general health, let's discuss how you can feed him to help decrease the inflammation and itching seen in allergic pets.

There is no one specific diet for the dog with atopic dermatitis. As a rule, pets with this condition do not have food allergies or hypersensitivities, so dietary therapy would seem at first glance not to be of any great benefit. Yet all holistic doctors can share stories of typically atopic pets who showed mild to moderate, and in some cases even great, improvement when fed a better, more natural diet. Certainly, pets with food allergies must be fed a hypoallergenic diet (see chapter 2, pages 43–46). It may be that the atopic pet showing less itching and inflammation when the diet is improved has some underlying food hypersensitivity that is resolved as the diet is improved. This may also explain the vast amount of improvement in the allergic pets that respond to nutritional supplements, which is the basis of the treatment I use for my allergic patients.

> Keep in mind that some dogs still itch on any commercial diet, even these better natural-style foods, while they show improvement when eating a homemade diet.

When possible, I recommend you switch to a homemade diet. This is the only way to ensure your complete control over the type and to some extent the quality of ingredients. If making a homemade diet is not practical, provide your dog a natural-style processed diet. Keep in mind that some dogs still itch on any commercial diet, even these better natural-style foods, while they show improvement when eating a homemade diet.

Sodium level is another element to consider. Doctors recommend that asthmatic people decrease their sodium intake because higher levels of dietary salt, common table salt, increase the reactivity of the bronchial passages to histamine, which causes breathing difficulties and even death. It is unknown how this plays out in allergic pets. However, most if not all prepared generic and even premium pet foods contain way too much sodium. Natural-style prepared foods do not seem to have this problem, but always check the label of the product to be sure. Pets with allergies would probably do well to eat a homemade low-sodium diet or natural-style prepared food without added salt.

If you suspect or have a diagnosis that your dog has food allergies, your doctor should prescribe a hypoallergenic diet with a novel protein source such as rabbit or venison (see chapter 2, page 43). I do not recommend feeding these unique protein sources to pets without food allergies. Not only are most of them quite expensive and difficult to obtain, if your dog develops food allergies to any of these unusual protein sources, your choices of what to feed at that point are severely limited.

## A Tip on Switching Diets

There is a secret to switching your pet to a new, healthier diet. Switching to the new food overnight may cause vomiting or diarrhea in a few dogs. Other pets are finicky and may not eat a new food that is suddenly introduced. The best way to offer your pet a new diet is by introducing it gradually. When you have about a week's worth of the old food remaining, purchase or prepare the new, healthier diet. Begin by adding about 10 percent of the new food to the previous food, and gradually increase the percentage until you run out of the old food and the pet is eating only the new diet. This trick usually prevents digestive problems and eases the transition to the new food.

# A HOMEMADE DIET
# FOR ADULT DOGS

Before feeding your pet a homemade diet, check with your doctor to make sure the diet does not compromise your pet's care. This recipe is a guideline only. You should determine the exact ingredients and amounts to feed in consultation with your veterinarian. The nutrient composition will vary depending upon the ingredients used. In general, this recipe supplies the daily nutritional and calorie needs for a 25- to 35-pound dog. The actual amount to feed will vary based upon the pet's weight. If the dog weighs more, feed more, if the dog weighs less, feed less.

---

3 large hard-boiled eggs *or* 1 cup of 2%-fat cottage cheese *or* ⅓ pound lean beef, poultry, lamb, venison or rabbit *or* ⅔ cup of tofu *or* 1 cup of cooked soybeans (Your doctor may adapt the specific protein source depending upon the severity of your dog's allergies.)

2 cups cooked long-grain brown rice *or* cooked noodles *or* ⅔ cup potatoes cooked with the skin

4 bonemeal tablets

1 multivitamin supplement

2 tablespoons canola oil

¼ teaspoon potassium chloride (salt substitute)

½ to 1 cup raw or steamed vegetables such as carrots, broccoli, etc. (optional)

---

*This recipe was adapted from *Prepared Dog and Cat Diets,* by Strombeck D. Home (Iowa State University Press, 1999), copyright 1999 Iowa State University Press. All Rights Reserved.

It may take some time to get your dog to accept the new diet. Additionally, it usually takes 4 to 8 weeks to see any positive effects, such as decreased itching and inflammation as the healthier diet allows his body to detoxify.

## Commercial Diets for Allergic Dogs

There are several commercial dog foods available for dogs with atopic dermatitis or food allergy dermatitis; some dogs have shown improvement when fed these special diets. These foods contain the "proper" ratio of omega-6 and omega-3 fatty acids or contain some of the novel protein sources discussed above. Since most commercial foods contain high levels of omega-6 fatty acids and low levels of omega-3 fatty acids, reversing this situation can increase the amount of omega-3 fatty acids in cell membranes and decrease itching in dogs.

> Good diet is important for general good health and in preventing the onset of allergies.

Some of these products use a new concept in diet involving "modified" proteins. Proteins can be chemically modified to make them smaller and less likely to cause an immune system reaction. This may be beneficial; however, your dog may be reacting to the by-products, fillers, and chemicals in commercial food as much as to the protein.

At first glance, these specially designed dog foods may seem like a good choice for the pet with allergies. There are some concerns for the holistic owner, however. While research seems to show that the proper ratio of omega-6 to omega-3 fatty acids is between 5:1 and 10:1, these special diets can still be less than healthy for the dog that requires natural foods. Just because the food is designed for an allergic or itchy dog doesn't mean it does not contain animal by-products, fillers, and various chemicals and artificial flavorings and preservatives.

Simply changing your dog's food from one commercially prepared food to another, even these special diets created for pets with allergies, won't usually resolve scratching. Switching a dog to a more natural diet (either homemade or natural-style packaged food), using a variety of supplements, shampooing and conditioning frequently, and occasionally employing conventional medical therapy in times of severe itching has proven beneficial for my patients; and the owners have not had to resort to the expensive "allergy" dog foods that are currently being promoted.

## Adding Supplements

Adding supplements to homemade dog food can be beneficial to the allergic dog if recommended by your veterinarian. Use only brand-name supplements and discuss all options with your veterinarian prior to giving them to your dog.

I recommend adding omega-3 fatty acids to homemade dog food, in addition to the canola oil. Follow the recommendations on the label of your omega-3 product, unless noted otherwise in the diet recipe. The omega-3 fatty acids can help decrease inflammation and itchiness.

Homemade dog food recipes often call for a calcium/phosphorus source, usually bonemeal as powder or tablets. As an alternative to bonemeal, you can use a natural product from Standard Process called Calcifood Wafers or Calcium Lactate. Use 1 Calcifood Wafer or 2 Calcium Lactate tablets for each ½ teaspoon of powdered bonemeal or 2 bonemeal tablets recommended in the recipe.

I also recommend a multivitamin-mineral supplement. You can use a natural raw (not chemically processed) human supplement, but keep in mind that each human supplement is recommended for the "average" 150-pound human. This means you should give a 50-pound dog ⅓ of the human supplement. A better suggestion is to use a natural product made for dogs such as Canine Plus (VetriScience); follow the dosage instructions on the label. I also like giving Catalyn, a natural vitamin-mineral supplement made by Standard Process (one tablet daily for dogs up to 30 pounds, two tablets for dogs from 30 to 60 pounds, and three tablets for dogs over 60 pounds). I use Catalyn in combination with Canine Plus for a synergistic effect. Your doctor may recommend other products as well.

Enzymes can help improve your dog's digestive efficiency with any diet, but especially with processed foods that do not contain natural digestive enzymes. Prozyme and Shake-n-Zyme are great plant enzyme products. Follow label directions.

You can provide additional phytonutrients and antioxidants by adding green food products containing barley grass, spirulina, or other super green foods to your dog's meal.

Good diet is important for general good health and in preventing the onset of allergies. By feeding your pet a more natural-style packaged food or homemade diet with the supplements I have recommended, you will lay the foundation for a complete program of holistic care for your allergic dog. This foundation along with the allergen avoidance techniques discussed in the next chapter can go a long way toward preventing outbreaks of allergic symptoms.

# CHAPTER SUMMARY

- Although diet alone cannot cure allergies, it can help prevent the onset of symptoms, and ease them when they occur.

- Overly processed packaged dog food is the least nutritious food to give your dog.

- Be aware of additives in processed packaged dog foods and read product labels carefully.

- Natural-style packaged dog foods, whether purchased in a store or from a veterinarian, are more nutritious than more processed foods.

- Homemade dog food can be simple to prepare and is the most nutritious for your dog.

- There is no substitute for a healthy lifestyle as a holistic healing approach.

# · 8 ·

# Avoiding Allergens

Y OU CAN'T KEEP your dog from having atopic dermatitis, but you can try to keep him from suffering the effects of the disease. Remember that the disease that causes
skin allergies is genetic and cannot be cured, but itchiness
and scratching won't occur unless foreign proteins, or allergens, trigger an allergic reaction. The best way to prevent
your dog from scratching due to allergies is to move some-
where like the desert or Alaska, where the chance of outdoor allergens is minimal! If that's not practical for you, do
the next best thing, and help your dog avoid the allergens
that cause him to itch. Once a skin test has determined his
exact allergen triggers, your prevention goal is to reduce his
allergen contact.

## MAINTAIN YOUR
## DOG'S ALLERGEN THRESHOLD

IF THE ALLERGENS are kept within your dog's allergen
threshold, he won't itch. Let's say for the illustration of this
concept that your pet is allergic to 30 different allergens. Let

us also suppose itching only occurs for him if 15 of these allergens are present together at the same time. This number is his allergen threshold. If he crosses it, he will itch. Let us say that 14 of his allergens are always present in his daily life. Your dog does not itch, since 15 allergens need to be present to cross his particular allergic threshold and cause him to itch. All winter your dog is fine. In the spring, ragweed blooms and provides the fifteenth allergen, so he itches. When spring ends and the ragweed is no longer releasing its highly allergenic pollens in your pet's environment, only 14 allergens are present and your pet, while still "allergic," no longer itches.

Now it's summer and flea season. A flea takes up residence on your pet and bites him. Your dog, like many pets with atopic dermatitis, is allergic to flea saliva. Now the flea becomes the fifteenth allergen your pet is exposed to, and the result is itching.

The concept of an allergen threshold is what makes it so important to minimize as many environmental allergens as possible, including parasites such as fleas. Every little bit you can do helps keep your dog's allergen load below his threshold.

# PRACTICE AVOIDANCE TECHNIQUES

THERE ARE METHODS for minimizing allergens in your pet's environment that don't require you to move to the frozen north or have your dog live in a bubble. There are actually some fairly simple steps you can take to reduce allergen contact.

Many pets are allergic to a variety of grasses, trees, pollens, and molds they come in contact with or inhale out-

doors. Often these pets are extremely itchy shortly after going outside and walking in the yard. To reduce contact with
these triggers, minimize outdoor time for your dog, especially during his allergic season (if one of his allergens is a
seasonally blooming plant).

Obviously, it is nearly impossible to keep a dog inside
all the time. But it helps to keep your dog indoors just after
you've watered the yard or just after you've cut the grass,
when allergens are active.
Consider putting booties
or a T-shirt on a severely
allergic pet when he does
go outdoors, and remov-
ing and washing them af-
ter he comes back inside.
You can also wash off his
feet with a wet washcloth
to remove some of the al-
lergens and thus reduce
his contact after he has
been outdoors.

> It helps to keep your
> dog indoors just after
> you've watered the
> yard or just after
> you've cut the grass,
> when allergens are
> active.

Even if your dog never goes outdoors, the allergens may
find him inside, tracked in by other pets and human household members. Frequently vacuuming and shampooing your
carpets reduces the foreign proteins that live deep in the
carpet fibers. Keeping all areas of your home clean of dust
helps as well. Window treatments, pillows, and upholstered
furniture can trap allergens just as carpets do. If your allergic
dog spends time in your car, you need to keep the carpet
and upholstery there clean as well.

Be especially vigilant about your dog's bedding. Change
and clean bedding frequently to decrease the allergenic
load. The most common allergen on the bedding is house

dust mites; frequent washing decreases the presence of this highly allergenic mite.

In addition to keeping the house, car, and bedding clean, you need to keep your dog clean as well. Frequently decontaminate your pet with a regimen of hypoallergenic shampooing and conditioning (see chapter 5, page 106). It is especially important to keep fleas and ticks off of your allergic pet. Remember that many allergic pets also have allergic reactions to fleas or other external (or internal) parasites. You must understand and appreciate that even one flea on a pet with atopic dermatitis is enough to make the pet itch, even after the flea is long gone!

> To keep your dog healthy and itch free, keep his environment smoke free.

You need to consider allergens in the air as well. To keep your indoor air free of them, change the air filters on your heating and air conditioning systems regularly. These filters trap the allergens, but if left in place too long, they will simply push the allergens back into the air. Better yet, use electrostatic or "allergy-free" air filters. High-efficiency particle-arresting (HEPA) filters can be attached to central air conditioning systems and are recommended for people and pets with allergies.

Cigarette smoke often acts as an allergen trigger in both people and animals. To keep your dog healthy and itch free, keep his environment smoke free. If you as an owner choose to smoke regularly in your pet's environment, not only can this exacerbate his allergies, but it also will increase his risk of respiratory disorders and lung cancer. If you choose to smoke, please do it outdoors to minimize further problems for your pet.

Make sure everyone in your household is aware of and understands your dog's allergies. Have everyone be on alert for the presence of seasonal allergens and fleas. Remind children who have just come in from playing outside to wash or change before playing with the allergic dog. Keep your allergy-free pets that go outdoors away from the allergic pet and the allergic pet's bedding. Find ways to provide exercise and stimulation for your allergic dog during periods when it must stay indoors.

By practicing all of the above avoidance techniques, you can help control your dog's allergies and keep him more comfortable.

# CHAPTER SUMMARY

- Since atopic dermatitis is a genetic disease, you can never cure a dog of it.

- You can prevent allergic reactions by reducing your dog's contact with his allergen triggers.

- Every dog has a threshold of how many allergens he can handle before a reaction occurs; keep within this threshold.

- Reduce your dog's outdoor time to reduce his contact with allergens.

- Keep your home clean, smoke free, and as free of allergens as possible.

- Wash your allergic pet and his bedding regularly to reduce contamination by allergens, fleas, and mites.

# ·9·

# Tying It All Together

A S WE COME to the end of this book, I hope I've given you a better understanding of atopic dermatitis. Remember, this is a genetic condition that can never be cured. However, you can find methods to lessen exposure to the allergens that trigger the allergic response and there are many treatment options to make your pet more comfortable and less prone to scratching.

Allergies may take months to properly treat with complementary therapies, as there is not "one" perfect therapy for every pet. Often your holistic veterinarian will need to try several therapies to determine which work best for your pet. Also keep in mind that the goal for most allergic pets is not to totally prevent any itching, but rather to keep your pet comfortably itchy most of the time. There are other causes of itching in pets in addition to allergic dermatitis, including mange, external and internal parasites, and other more serious problems. Therefore, a proper diagnosis is essential before choosing any therapy.

While conventional medications such as corticosteroids and antihistamines do have their place in the treatment of some allergic pets, there are too many potential side effects from these drugs, particularly corticosteroids, to use them as the sole, long term therapy for all but the very few pets that do not improve with any other treatment.

Complementary therapies such as nutritional supplements, dietary therapy, acupuncture, herbal therapy, and homeopathy all have their place in the treatment of the pet with atopic dermatitis. Often they can serve as the sole therapy, although many times your doctor may combine them with lower doses of conventional medications to help your dog.

To tie all this together, here is my holistic approach to the allergic pet:

- Provide your dog a healthy life. Feed your pet a nutritious diet from puppyhood and practice an exercise program suited for your size dog.

- Establish a relationship with a holistic veterinarian for the regular care of your pet. All approaches are more successful when the dog is comfortable with medical procedures and the vet is acquainted with the dog.

- Once you see that your dog is scratching, obtain a correct diagnosis as soon as possible. Because allergies can make your dog terribly uncomfortable and susceptible to chronic skin infections, the sooner you start complementary therapies to make the pet feel better the better for the pet.

- While atopic dermatitis is the most common cause of scratching, there are other causes. Some of these are opportunistic conditions that are secondary to the allergic condition. Others are separate conditions completely. Some of these causes are very serious diseases.

- Proper diagnostic testing is needed to rule out other causes of scratching. This usually involves skin scrapings, skin cytology, fungal cultures, skin biopsies, skin cultures, and blood testing.

- If your pet is diagnosed with allergic dermatitis, discuss the numerous treatment options with your veterinarian. Pets that are severely itchy are often provided with traditional medical treatments, such as short-term low doses of corticosteroids or antihistamines, to give quick relief. Since most complementary therapies, especially dietary therapy and nutritional supplements take 1 to 2 months or more to "kick in," conventional medical treatments may be needed for short-term relief.

- Practice prevention techniques for avoiding allergens.

- Give your dog frequent baths and conditioning with hypoallergenic products as these can often decrease the need for both conventional and other complementary approaches.

- If necessary and suggested by your veterinarian, use dietary therapy and nutritional and other supplements.

- Use acupuncture and/or homeopathy as needed. If nutritional therapies don't give the desired results, keep the pet on the products to improve their overall nutritional health but use acupuncture and/or homeopathy to aid in decreasing inflammation and itching and stimulate the pet's immune system.

# LONG-TERM APPROACHES

FOR LONG-TERM THERAPY, most of my patients can be successfully maintained without side effects on a regime of nutritional supplements using products containing omega-3 fatty acids and raw food and glandular supplements plus bathing and condition 2 to 3 times per week or daily during their most itchy seasons. Occasionally I add homeopathy, acupuncture, or conventional medications if the pet is having a "bad day."

Every doctor develops his favorite approach to dealing with various disorders such as atopic dermatitis. In order to treat the pet holistically, it's important to try to do what's best for the pet's overall health and well-being. The pet must be treated humanely and you must stay involved in treatment decisions for your pets.

There is no hard and fast rule I use when deciding what approach is best for a particular patient. I explain options to the owners, including side effects and costs of the treatments. In working with owners, I like to form a team whose goal is to do what's best for the pet. When owners are involved, they are more likely to take an interest in the therapy. Additionally, they feel important to the pet's outcome and are a vital member of the treatment team. This is a far different approach from the doctor who sees himself as "God" and uses "shotgun" therapy with no owner involvement. Pet owners are loving, dedicated, kind-hearted people. It is essential that they be involved in the decision-making process, as they are ultimately responsible for their pets.

> It is essential that owners be involved in the decision-making process, as they are ultimately responsible for their pets.

# BIBLIOGRAPHY

For more information about holistic pet care for pets, or to find a holistic veterinarian in your area, contact the American Holistic Veterinary Medical Association at 410-569-0795 and visit the Pet Care Naturally Web site at www.petcarenaturally.com.

Ackerman, L. "Dermatologic Uses of Fatty Acids in Dogs and Cats." *Veterinary Medicine* (December 1995): 1149–1155.

Ackerman, L. "Nondermatologic Indications for Fatty Acid Supplementation in Dogs and Cats." *Veterinary Medicine* (December 1995): 1156–1159.

Ackerman, L. "Reviewing the Biochemical Properties of Fatty Acids." *Veterinary Medicine* (December 1995): 1138–1148.

Altman, S. "Small Animal Acupuncture: Scientific Basis and Clinical Applications." In *Complementary and Alternative Veterinary Medicine,* edited by A. Schoen and S. Wynn. Philadelphia, PA: W.B. Saunders, 1999: 147–168.

Balch, J., and P. Balch. *Prescription for Nutritional Healing.* Garden City, NY: Avery, 1997: 110–122.

Belfield, W. "Orthomolecular Medicine: A Practitioner's Perspective." In *Complementary and Alternative Veterinary Medicine,* edited by A. Schoen and S. Wynn. Philadelphia, PA: W.B. Saunders, 1999: 113–132.

Bratman, S., and D. Kroll. *Natural Health Bible.* Rocklin, CA: Prima, 1999: 3–4, 66–68.

Chen, J. *Clinical Manual of Oriental Medicine.* La Puente, CA: The Lotus Collection, 1999.

Day, C. *The Homeopathic Treatment of Small Animals: Principles and Practice.* Essex, Britain: C.W. Daniel, 1990: 96–100.

Day, C. "Veterinary Homeopathy: Principles and Practice." In *Complementary and Alternative Veterinary Medicine,* edited by A. Schoen and S. Wynn. Philadelphia, PA: W.B. Saunders, 1999: 485–514.

DeBoer, D. "Management of Chronic and Recurrent Pyoderma in the Dog." In *Kirk's Current Veterinary Therapy XII: Small Animal Practice,* edited by John Bonagura. Philadelphia, PA: W.B. Saunders, 1995: 413–415.

DeCava, J. "Glandular Supplements." *Nutrition News and Views* (May/June 1997), P.O. Box 877, West Barnstable, MA 02668-0877.

DeGroot, J. "Veterinary Medical Uses and Sources of Omega-3 Fatty Acids." *Veterinary Forum* (May 1998): 42–48.

DeGuzman, E. "Western Herbal Medicine: Clinical Applications." In *Complementary and Alternative Veterinary Medicine,* edited by A. Schoen and S. Wynn. Philadelphia, PA: W.B. Saunders, 1999: 337–378.

Greco, D., and E. Behrend. "Corticosteroid Withdrawal Syndrome." In *Kirk's Current Veterinary Therapy XII: Small Animal Practice,* edited by John Bonagura. Philadelphia, PA: W.B. Saunders, 1995: 413–415.

Hannah, S. "Nutritional Considerations for Food Allergies in Dogs: Nutritional Management Based on the Principles of Food Hypersensitivity." *Purina Owner's Guide,* 1997.

Hodgson, J. "Capitalizing on Carbohydrates." *Bio/Technology* 8 (February 1990): 109–111.

Hodgson, J. "Capitalizing on Carbohydrates." *Bio/Technology* 9 (July 1991): 609–613.

Ihrke, P. "Pruritus." In *Textbook of Veterinary Internal Medicine,* Vol. I, edited by S. Ettinger and E. Feldman. Philadelphia, PA: W.B. Saunders, 1999: 31-36.

Kwochka, K. "Shampoo and Moisturizing Rinses in Veterinary Dermatology." In *Kirk's Current Veterinary Therapy XII: Small Animal Practice,* edited by John Bonagura. Philadelphia, PA: W.B. Saunders, 1995: 611-617.

Ledford, D. "Urticaria and Angioedema." In *Allergic Diseases, Diagnosis and Treatment,* edited by P. Lieberman and J. Anderson. Totowa, NJ: Humana Press, 1997: 189-204.

Lininger Jr., S., A. Gaby, S. Austin, D. Brown, J. Wright, and A. Duncan. *The Natural Pharmacy.* 2d ed. Rocklin, CA: Prima, 1999, 15-16, 64-65, 76-77.

MacDonald, J. "Glucocorticoid Therapy." In *Textbook of Veterinary Internal Medicine,* Vol. I, edited by S. Ettinger and E. Feldman. Philadelphia, PA: W.B. Saunders, 1999: 307-317.

McKeever, P., and H. Globus. "Canine Otitis Externa." In *Kirk's Current Veterinary Therapy XII: Small Animal Practice,* edited by John Bonagura. Philadelphia, PA: W.B. Saunders, 1995: 647-655.

Macleod, G. *Dogs: Homeopathic Remedies.* Essex, Britain: C.W. Daniel, 1994: 98-116.

Miller Jr., W. "Treatment of Generalized Demodicosis in Dogs." In *Kirk's Current Veterinary Therapy XII: Small Animal Practice,* edited by John Bonagura. Philadelphia, PA: W.B. Saunders, 1995: 625-628.

Moore, M. "Skin Allergy Agent." *Veterinary Forum* (October 1999): 26.

Murray, M., and J. Pizzorno. *Encyclopedia of Natural Medicine.* 2d ed. Rocklin, CA: Prima, 1998: 260-272, 448-454, 464-475.

Pitcairn, R., and S. Pitcairn. *Dr. Pitcairn's Complete Guide to Natural Health for Dogs and Cats.* Emmaus, PA: Rodale Press, 1995: 229-232, 303-308.

Plumb, D. *Veterinary Drug Handbook.* 3d ed. Ames, IA: Iowa State University Press, 1999: 214–216, 306–309, 333–334.

Purina. "Meeting the Special Nutritional Needs of Dogs with Food Allergies." *Purina CNM Owner's Guide,* 1997.

Reinhart, G. "Review of Omega-3 Fatty Acids and Dietary Influences on Tissue Concentrations." Proceedings of the 1996 IAMS International Nutritional Symposium, 235–242.

Reinhart, G., D. Scott, and Wm. Miller Jr. "A Controlled Dietary Omega-6:Omega-3 Ratio Reduces Pruritus in Non-Food Allergic Dogs." Proceedings of the 1996 IAMS International Nutritional Symposium, 277–284.

Schick, M., R. Schick, and G. Reinhart. "The Role of Polyunsaturated Fatty Acids in the Canine Epidermis: Normal Structural and Functional Components, Inflammatory Disease State Components, and as Therapeutic Dietary Components." Proceedings of the 1996 IAMS International Nutritional Symposium, 267–276.

Schultz, K. "The Current Immunology of Allergy." In *Kirk's Current Veterinary Therapy XII: Small Animal Practice,* edited by John Bonagura. Philadelphia, PA: W.B. Saunders, 1995: 628–630.

Schwartz, C. "Chinese Herbal Medicine in Small Animal Practice." In *Complementary and Alternative Veterinary Medicine,* edited by A. Schoen and S. Wynn. Philadelphia, PA: W.B. Saunders, 1999: 437–450.

Scott, D. "Rational Use of Glucocorticoids in Dermatology." In *Kirk's Current Veterinary Therapy XII: Small Animal Practice,* edited by John Bonagura and J. Kirk. Philadelphia, PA: W.B. Saunders, 1995: 573–581.

Scott, D., W. Miller Jr., and C. Griffin. *Muller and Kirk's Small Animal Dermatology.* 5th ed. Philadelphia, PA: W.B. Saunders, 1995.

Smith Jr., F.W.K. "The Neurophysiologic Basis of Acupuncture." In *Veterinary Acupuncture: Ancient Art to Modern Medicine,* edited by A. Schoen. Philadelphia, PA: W.B. Saunders, 1994: 33–54.

Strombeck, D. *Home-Prepared Dog and Cat Diets.* Ames, IA: Iowa State University Press, 1999: 127–216.

Tilford, G., and M. Wulff-Tilford. *All You Ever Wanted to Know about Herbs for Pets.* Irvine CA: BowTie Press, 1999: 335–346.

Ullman, D. "Homeopathic Medicine: Principles and Practice." In *Complementary and Alternative Veterinary Medicine,* edited by A. Schoen and S. Wynn. Philadelphia, PA: W.B. Saunders, 1999: 469–484.

Vaughn, D., and G. Reinhart. "Influence of Dietary Fatty Acid Ratios on Tissue Eicosanoid Production and Blood Coagulation Parameters in Dogs." Proceedings of the 1996 IAMS International Nutritional Symposium, 243–246.

Waters, K.C. "Acupuncture for Dermatologic Disorders in Dogs and Cats." In *Veterinary Acupuncture: Ancient Art to Modern Medicine,* edited by A. Schoen. Philadelphia, PA: W.B. Saunders, 1994: 269–276.

Whitaker, J. *Dr. Whitaker's Guide to Natural Healing.* Rocklin, CA: Prima Publishing, 1996: 163–171, 239–241.

# INDEX